TANDEM COUPLES COUNSELING

This book introduces the protocol known as Tandem Couples Counseling (TCC), a ground-breaking model that provides sound theoretical explanations and interventions that address the inherent difficulties in traditional forms of couples counseling.

Tandem Couples Counseling: An Innovative Approach to Working with High Conflict Couples synthesizes the research literature from the fields of couples counseling and group work into a compelling therapeutic approach. Extensive case examples illuminate the dynamics and skills of the approach. Assessment processes and rich descriptions of the treatment protocols are included, enabling integration, and understanding of how to implement this approach with clients as well as immediately work to improve the connection in existing co-therapy arrangements.

The text is an essential guide for counseling professionals on how to build, maintain, and use the co-therapy relationship as an agent of change in high-conflict couples.

Justin E. Levitov, Ph.D., LPC, is a professor emeritus at Loyola University New Orleans, USA.

Kevin A. Fall, Ph.D., LPC-S, is a professor and chair of the Department of Counseling, Leadership, Adult Education, and School Psychology at Texas State University, USA.

TANDEM COUPLES COUNSELING

An Innovative Approach to Working with High Conflict Couples

Justin E. Levitov and Kevin A. Fall

Routledge
Taylor & Francis Group

NEW YORK AND LONDON

First published 2021
by Routledge
52 Vanderbilt Avenue, New York, NY 10017

and by Routledge
2 Park Square, Milton Park, Abingdon, Oxon, OX14 4RN

Routledge is an imprint of the Taylor & Francis Group, an informa business

Library of Congress Cataloging-in-Publication Data
A catalog record for this title has been requested

ISBN: 978-0-367-22429-5 (hbk)
ISBN: 978-0-367-22430-1 (pbk)
ISBN: 978-0-429-27896-9 (ebk)

Typeset in Joanna
by MPS Limited, Dehradun

This book is dedicated to the memory of Dr. William "Bill" Rosenbaum, cherished friend, colleague, and unwavering fan of Tandem Couples Counseling. You inspired so many people to become great counselors. Thank you.

CONTENTS

PREFACE

We remain impressed to this very day by what a privilege it is to enter into the life of a couple as they struggle with the distress, disappointment, and emotional pain of conflict replacing what once was love, joy, and enthusiasm for a future together. While couples work is an interesting and highly rewarding profession, it is also a rare and precious opportunity to help families heal. The journey to health can be quite difficult: it can bring to surface complicated life experiences—feelings of shame, embarrassment, and regret; it can ask people to own up behaviors, thoughts, and ideas that have been hurtful to themselves and to those they love; and it can also open new ways of sharing life's burdens and joys that simply were not available before therapy.

Early on, we wanted to honor the people who allowed us to help them in a way that provides the proper environment and level of respect for their relationship. We developed an interest and local "specialty" for treating couples who have experienced a considerable number of failures in previous counseling sessions. Like our colleagues, we attempted to help them in the traditional one counselor-two clients setting, but we were hit with the same obstacles as the previous treatments. It was for this reason that we opted to take a fresh look at the process of counseling and do our best to refocus our efforts. While doing traditional couples counseling, we saw alarming flaws—even seemingly well-meaning efforts—that hindered the clients' attempts to improve their relationship. To overcome these problems, we decided to pivot our focus and direct our activities in what we hoped would be better ways.

This book details our efforts to make the couple's relationship the singular focus of our work. We have heard, "how can I get my needs met?" or "what needs to happen for my partner to do this?" for too long. Often, we hear about how great everything would be if their partner thinks the way they do; we know these discussions lead nowhere and the couple remains as unhappy and conflicted as they were before therapy. Eventually, we decided to shift our efforts and see the Relationship as our client; we replaced questions concerning each of the couples with those relevant to their relationship. These preliminary efforts uncovered a new and immensely valuable therapeutic focus: intimacy. By focusing on the relationship, we began to understand how people can crave and fear intimacy at the same time. Our clients were open and motivated—they share the distorted and ineffective models of intimacy they've been exposed to and explain how they assumed that sexual intimacy was all a couple needed. They explored their earliest family experiences, offering one dysfunctional model of intimacy after another handed down by people they loved and respected and who loved and respected them. Even in so much distress, they continued to share their experiences to find ways to help build the intimacy that was missing in their lives—injuring them and their relationship every day.

We developed new methods and strategies and invited our clients to work with us to assess their usefulness. Our concerns quickly vanished once we saw how our clients welcomed the new interventions with enthusiasm. We learned that the respect we show them as their therapists impacts the way they respect each other. The couples were eager to learn about our relationship patterns—how we, as therapists, manage our differences as we struggle to produce decisions. A special kind of cooperation developed between us that produced healing qualities in and of itself. Inspired, we continue to further explore the phenomena and develop new ways of harnessing its power.

This book is the culmination of over 20 years of work with what we call Tandem Couples Counseling (TCC). We aspire to provide some guidance to mental health professionals who may want to incorporate these ideas into their work. The book is filled with case samples and illustrations pulled from common patterns and themes that have emerged in our supervision of TCC cases for over two decades. The names and identifying information are changed to honor confidentiality. We hope that this book will be the beginning of your relationship with TCC and that it encourages you to create more ideas on how to best help couples in need.

None of these accomplishments could have been possible without the dedicated support of great colleagues and motivated clients. We are grateful to Dr. Trudie Atkinson, for her early work in Tandem Couples Counseling. She offered wise and incisive guidance, useful suggestions, and encouragement at an early and critical point in the development of this model. The staff at Trinity Counseling and Training took a great interest in our work from the outset and we thank them for creating a space for us to share our methods—for their willingness to have students and staff use approaches we have developed. Family Services of Greater New Orleans also adopted our model to use with select couple's cases. We are especially thankful to so many of our students—their excitement about what we're doing was contagious, motivating, and inspiring. One student in particular—Bill Rosenbaum—a highly-respected New Orleans counselor, made no secret of his respect for Tandem Couples Counseling. He had been asking for this book for more than a decade. Sadly, he passed away before it was published; however, we think and hope that he somehow knew his request would eventually be granted.

We are also grateful to our families. Books require an inordinate amount of time, to say nothing of the time commitment warranted to develop new couples counseling methods; however, it was a far greater gift they offered than that of time. Our families taught us that successful, respectful, loving, and intimate couple relationships were indeed possible. Our families also showed us that it is not enough to create successful relationships – it is equally important to help others achieve the same results.

Finally, to all the couples who came with us on this journey: thank you! You have no idea how much we deeply appreciate you for allowing us into your family and couple life, how grateful we are for your honesty, and how pleased we are to have our relationship relate to yours. We have been careful with regards to your anonymity, but you know who you are and hopefully, you'll recognize how much we appreciate you for being amazing people.

1

A BRIEF HISTORY OF COUPLES COUNSELING AND THE EVOLUTION OF TANDEM COUPLES COUNSELING

Context is key. How many times have you sat with a new couple in counseling and asked them to tell you the story of their relationship? How and why something came into being is seen as useful to the true understanding of that object, so we thought discussing how and why Tandem Couples Counseling (TCC) was developed would be a good way of providing context for what is in this book. You will get the particulars later, the phases, and the techniques. For now, prepare for a history lesson—both TCC and that of couples' treatment. We will begin with some insight into the origins of TCC.

TCC was an experimental protocol that we developed 20 years ago. In a word, we were frustrated with inconsistent results when we saw couples in the usual one counselor-two client setting. We also identified a growing number of couples for whom traditional approaches tended to have limited efficacy, and worried that some efforts could worsen their struggle. With these concerns in mind, we began to try diverse ways of doing couples counseling. Enough counseling theories existed on which to base interventions, but how the therapy should be conducted seemed a fertile place to begin improvement. I (J.E.L.) remember the moment that provided the catalyst for some of the ideas outlined in this book:

I was sitting with a new couple, eagerly anticipating the beginning of a new therapeutic journey. To begin, I prepared to do what I normally do in the preliminary stages of counseling: build rapport, gather information, and orient the clients to the culture of counseling. The couple immediately started angrily yelling at one another, blaming each other for every struggle they had endured in their 10-year relationship. I had seen this before; I intervened by gently stopping the melee and encouraging them to listen and try to understand what the other person was saying. I asserted that both would get time to share their perspectives. Instead of settling into the process, the couple attacked each other more aggressively. I intervened again, patiently pointing out the pattern that was emerging and deftly pointing out that they were recreating the behaviors that were contributing to the problems in their relationship; however, nothing seems to help or redirect them. I asked them to reflect on the session before we ended for the day. They each said they felt worse and that even though they had been to counsel on and off for years, it did not seem to help. I consulted and tried for three more sessions but to no avail. My colleagues offered advice such as, "[s]ome people aren't ready for change," "[d]efeating counselors sounds like the couple's way of bonding," and several wanted to "fire the couple." As I reflected on this case and talked to colleagues, I came to realize that this couple isn't alone and I began to explore how to modify the traditional couples counseling approach to meet the needs of these exceptional clients.

As clinicians, we realize early in our practice that, while clients come and go, couples tended to remain in our minds for months, even years later. We fully understand that our work with couples greatly influences their families and that the stakes are often quite high—their children's health and well-being often hung in the balance, as well as their relationships with family, friends, and coworkers. Working with couples is both intrinsically interesting and particularly important.

Even in our early years, we believed that if couples work was done well it could benefit not only the couple but a wide range of related people as well. In short, TCC evolved to help couples that seem to be beyond help.

With that brief background and personal introduction in mind, we move to provide a limited overview of the history of couples counseling. We hope that by understanding the foundation and course of the field of the couple's work, the rationale for TCC will be clearer as we move through the book.

A Brief History of Couples Counseling

Couples counseling has enjoyed a long and rich history. The earliest mention we can find of the practice of couples counseling was in 1929 when Abraham and Hannah Stone established the Marriage Consultation Center in New York. This was followed by the Marriage Council of Philadelphia founded by Emily Mudd in 1932, Paul Popenoe's American Institute of Family Relations in 1939, and the American Association of Marriage Counselors in 1942. Since these humble beginnings, couples counseling has been firmly rooted in the therapeutic landscape across the globe.

While this book intends to elucidate a specific application of couples counseling, we think it is important to understand the foundations of the modality so the reader can discern overlaps and deviation from the standard practice. Specifically, we wanted to trace the history and show some distinctions between what traditional couples counseling offers and how TCC provides an alternative to the standard, two clients, one counselor format. It is beyond the scope of the book to provide a detailed account of the history, and readers who are wanting more can consult (Capuzzi & Stauffer, 2015; Gladding, 2018; Gurman & Fraenkel, 2002; Gurman, Lebow, & Snyder, 2015).

On its surface, the idea and benefit of offering counseling to couples counseling seem self-evident. If a couple is productive and emotionally healthy and sound, it stands that the family will also benefit. It makes sense that throughout the last 90 years, counseling and psychotherapy theory and practice have been applied to help troubled couples and by extension troubled families. According to Paterson (2009):

> Society has long recognized the positive impact that a steadfast adult relationship can have—not only on the individuals who have united to form a couple but also on the emotional health of those in the couple's sphere of influence. These relationships help define us and, some say, strengthen our society.

Gurman and Fraenkel's (2002) history of couples counseling is the most complete and comprehensive review currently available, albeit 20 years old at this point. The authors meticulously document decades of theoretical and clinical changes. Couples counseling, like all other mental health applications, has been heavily influenced by changes in counseling theory, the creation of various mental health professions (Mental Health Counselors, Marriage and Sex Therapists, Family Therapists, Psychologists, and Social Workers), and the powerful social changes that occurred. Gurman and Fraenkel (2002, p. 204) offer a four-stage model for exploring the evolution of couples counseling below:

Atheoretical Marriage Counseling Formation (1930–1963): This stage is marked by the beginnings of the profession of marriage counselors—a wellness-oriented group of individuals who focus on psychoeducation and prevention. It is also interesting to note that in this phase, it is highly unusual for the couple to receive treatment conjointly (together, in the same room). Olson (1970) noted that it wasn't until the end of the 1960s that couples' counselors utilized the conjoint method of treatment; Gurman and Fraenkel commented that it took the influence of psychoanalysis to push through with this approach.

Psychoanalytic Experimentation and Reemergence (1931–1966; 1985–present): As clergy and social workers developed their prevention-based approach to marital issues, psychiatrists used psychoanalysis to treat problems associated with intimacy and marriage. It is in this experimentation phase that concurrent, combined, collaborative, and collaborative combined treatment approaches emerged. We will explore each one as they are precursors to the TCC approach.

Concurrent treatment is when a couple is seen individually by the same therapist. In these early days, the analyst treats each of the couples individually, but at the same time. The original psychoanalytic assumption maintained that one should help the other, or both couples, with their psychological issues, and over time the couple relationship would eventually benefit. Prochaska and Prochaska (1978) outlined how Mittelman (1948) was the first to articulate the concurrent approach when dealing with marital problems. According to Prochaska and Prochaska (1978), "Concurrent analysis was aimed at each spouse developing insight into the particular neurotic needs that he or she brought into the marriage. With the development of insight in each spouse separately, they could begin to change the way they saw each other and to relate on a more mature rather than infantile level (p. 13)." It is again important to note that this form of treatment is done without the couple being in the same room. The notion of the couple working together in treatment was viewed as extremely problematic and disruptive to the transference process.

While eventually, couples began to be seen conjointly (Sager, 1967), it is hard to imagine why it took so long to bring both into the same office. Methods and techniques for seeing a couple together were offensive under psychoanalysis, and it had to wait until the theory expanded or developed another modality—such as group counseling—to provide the conceptual base for seeing multiple clients at a time. Without this growth, clinicians were bound by their philosophical paradigm; cultural values must change to permit the use or consideration of various techniques. In earlier days, meeting with a couple could have been deemed presumptuous, improper, or even too risky for both parties. Couples were often left under the care of clergy or revered older family member, and the very idea of talking to someone outside of the family about marital problems would be forbidden. In the end, couples were left to explore relational change as individuals, and even that was an innovation.

While concurrent treatment was controversial in the psychoanalytic community for its inclusion and consideration of relational issues, it remained the popular form of treatment for marital issues until conjoint marital therapy became the primary approach in the late 1960s. As the experimentation phase progressed, several other forms of marital counseling were attempted. *Combined marital therapy* (Greene & Solomon, 1963) involved one therapist who saw the couple in individual and conjoint sessions. *Collaborative therapy* (Martin & Bird, 1963) utilized two counselors who saw the couple individually (one counselor per individual) and then consulted on the treatment. *Collaborative combined* treatment (Royce & Hogan, 1960), the closest match to TCC, assigned separate counselors for each individual and then the four would meet for conjoint sessions. What an amazing time of innovation the late 1960s must have been in the field of couples counseling!

This shift to meeting and working with the couple together in any of the above forms was a true innovation and was highly controversial to the dominant psychoanalytic tradition. Gurman and Fraenkel (2002) assert that the move to conjoint treatment was "revolutionary" (p. 210) and cleared a space for ideas that moved beyond the individual. This new way of thinking combined with the widespread use of conjoint counseling for the treatment of couples' issues in the 1960s, also paved the way for the next large growth in couples counseling.

Family Therapy Incorporation (1963–1985)

Though the psychoanalytic theory was the first to be used to help couples, several counseling theories have been adapted for use with couples and families over the ever-evolving history of counseling. The most profound shift during this phase came with the arrival of General Systems Theory. Systems Theory offered yet another useful perspective, one where the emphasis was on the family system rather than the individuals. This approach allows therapists to see the structures that families live in and offer useful methods to improve the conditions for all members of the family, especially the couple. By understanding the role anxiety plays within the family and illustrating how members of the family participate in the healthy and unhealthy management of that anxiety, couple's counselors have a structural focus from which to work.

Systems Theory also helps couple's counselors understand and accept a particularly important reality: people establish relationships with others who have about the same level of "differentiation," according to Kerr and Bowen (1988). While a couple may appear overtly quite different from one another emotionally, socially, or intellectually they are equally matched on the differentiation scales. For example, highly differentiated individuals form and maintain relationships with other highly differentiated people. This is important because even though one member of the couple may externally look more maladaptive, both are functioning at about the same level. By keeping this in mind, a therapist's tendency to see one person as healthier and the other as needing is properly mitigated.

Systems Theory also helps the couple's therapists remain mindful of the relationship and how it manifests itself between the couple and within the family. The concept of triangulation helps make this point and offers counselors a tool for reducing conflict. Kerr and Bowen (1988) point out that triangulation occurs in all relationships—create tension between any two people and a third person will be brought in to try and reduce the tension. The authors saw this as so fundamental that even lower life forms in the animal kingdom relied upon it to reduce anxiety. Triangulation is not limited to individuals within the structure of the family—unfortunately, counselors are usually triangulated unwittingly, and at times destructively, into their clients' couple relationship. Such triangulations occur in both obvious and more hidden ways. Skilled couple's counselors continuously estimate the risk of triangulation with every intervention they pursue as they seek to "help" the couple.

While it might be interesting to know that there was a time when the fields of marriage counseling and family counseling were separate entities, the fields are fairly indistinguishable from one another now—training and professional organizations are comfortably intertwined. Each counseling theory emphasizes a different perspective from which to help and to view relationship struggles, the theories when taken together offer a panoramic view of how best to understand a couple's conflicts and methods to improve their relationship. Table 1.1. gives you a broad sense of some of the major theories under the Systems Theory umbrella. These theories represent much of the foundation of today's marriage and family profession and these roots have continued into the next and last phase.

Refinement, Extension, Diversification, & Integration (1985-present): The last phase is characterized by a profession that continues to grow and embed itself in the world of mental health. While psychodynamic approaches continue to have some influence, other theories have become increasingly popular over the past two decades. Behavioral Marital Therapy (BMT; Stuart, 1980), Emotionally Focused Therapy (EFT; Johnson, 1996), and the Gottman approach (1994, 1999) are three of

Table 1.1 Comparison Chart of Major System's Approaches

Name of Founder / Name of Therapy	Murray Bowen / Multigenerational Therapy	James Framo / Object-Relations Therapy	Ivan Boszormnenyi-Nagy / Contextual Therapy
View of system	A system is an emotional unit—a network of interlocking relationships—best understood when viewed from a multigenerational framework.	The system is an intricate system with its own unique bonding, rules, homeostatic mechanisms, secret alliances, communication network, myths, regressive features, and dynamic influences from previous generations.	The system understanding is based on the principle of "reciprocity," having received and having to reciprocate. Each spouse brings the heritage and loyalties of previous generations into the context of the new system.
The healthy system	Intellect characterized by emotional detachment is the hallmark of the healthy system. Members have learned to establish their own identities, to differentiate themselves from the system of origin.	In the healthy systems: parents are well-differentiated, generational boundaries are clear, the loyalty of the spouses is greater to the system of procreation than the system of origin, spouses view the marital subsystem as primary, and autonomy for all system members are encouraged.	Spouses who experienced a high degree of relational equitability in the families of origin bring to the marriage a ledger of indebtedness and entitlements that are balanced. Thus, they can focus on the mutual welfare interests of the entire system.
Dysfunction	Members of the marital dyad have poor differentiation of self and are emotionally "stuck-together" to their	Intrapsychic conflicts derived from the system of origin are replicated with spouse and/or children. Efforts at	Dysfunction occurs when the adult child is not able to transfer loyalty from

	families of origin. Styles of origin are repeated in marital relationships and are passed on to children.	the interpersonal resolution of the inner conflict are at the heart of the kinds of distress found in troubled couples and families.	the system of origin to the new marital relationship; loyalty owed to previous/subsequent generations conflict with loyalty owed to spouse, siblings, friends, and peers.
Role of therapist	The therapist is a "coach"—an active expert who educates system members (primarily the marital dyad) but remains disengaged from the system: detached, objective, and neutral.	The therapist is active and very structured, moving from empathy to confrontation. The therapist usually works with a co-therapist who is of the other gender. The therapist works primarily with the marital dyad only and has a strong "educative" function.	The therapist is an active, encouraging guide. Using "multidirectional partiality" he/she is an advocate for all persons involved in therapy, moving from gentle exploration to a more confronting style while holding participants responsible for their own movement.
Goal of therapy	The basic overarching goal is to assist system members—primarily the marital dyad—toward a better level of differentiation of self. Growth in differentiation will facilitate the	The two major goals for each member of the marital dyad are: (1) to discover what issues/agendas from the system of origin impact the current system, and (2) to have a	The goal is to enable participants to move toward relational integrity, relational commitments, and

(Continued)

Table 1.1 (Continued)

Name of Founder Name of Therapy	Murray Bowen Multigenerational Therapy	James Framo Object-Relations Therapy	Ivan Boszormnenyi-Nagy Contextual Therapy
	reduction of anxiety and relief from symptoms.	corrective experience with parents and siblings from the system of origin.	balances of fairness, and to enable system members to gain trust in one another's increasingly trustworthy input.
Primary techniques	Genograms, therapist detachment as a primary technique, defining the roles/relationships in the system, teaching the **"I"** position, defusing emotion and avoiding blame, examining/reestablishing contact with the system of origin.	Male-female therapy team; standard techniques of *Couples Therapy; Couples Group Therapy; System of Origin Sessions*—bringing in the system of origin with individual members of the marital dyad to deal directly with unresolved attachment issues.	Three-generational assessment, conjoint system therapy as the norm, multidirectional partiality, self-disclosure, guiding, confrontation, instruction in building trusting and equitable relationships, suggestions, directives, loyalty framing, exoneration, some use of co-therapy.

Name of Founder **Name of Therapy** View of system	**Virginia Satir** **Process/Communications Approach** Systems are balanced, rule-governed and through the basic components of communication and self-esteem,	**Jay Haley** **Strategic Therapy** The system involves power relations and has rules by which it operates. The power struggle is not a question of who controls whom but

	provide a context for growth and development.	of who controls the definition of the relationship and by what maneuvers.
The healthy system	In the healthy system, members are in touch with their own feelings, communicate in a congruent manner, accept others as different from themselves, and view those differences as a chance to learn and explore rather than as a threat.	Functional families develop suitable up-front methods of dealing with conflict/control struggles. In addition, they have clear rules and a balance of stability and flexibility.
Dysfunction	Dysfunctional systems consist of persons whose freedom to grow and develop has been blocked. Dysfunctional behavior results from the interplay of low self-esteem, incongruent communication, poor system functioning, and dysfunctional system rules (both overt and covert).	Symptoms are understood as an attempt to control a relationship. The maneuver to control is understood as dysfunctional if one or both participants deny the issue of control and/or exhibit symptomatic behavior in the process of doing so.
Role of therapist	The therapist is a facilitator, a resource person, an observer, a detective, and a teacher/model of congruent communication and warmth and empathy. The therapist is highly active, personally involved in the	The therapist takes an active, directive, and authoritative "take-charge" approach to the power struggle that is therapy. The therapist assumes the role of the system change-maker; he/she

(Continued)

Table 1.1 (Continued)

Name of Founder / Name of Therapy	Murray Bowen Multigenerational Therapy	James Framo Object-Relations Therapy	Ivan Boszormnenyi-Nagy Contextual Therapy
Goal of therapy	system yet able to confront when necessary. Three overarching goals: each system member will (1) grow in understanding of self and in the ability to communicate congruently, (2) increase respect for the uniqueness of each system member, and (3) view individual uniqueness as an opportunity for growth.	assumes temporary leadership of the system. Change in the system is the basic goal of therapy. Therapy is focused on altering behavior patterns maintaining the presenting problem.	
Primary techniques	System life chronology, conjoint system therapy is the norm (marital dyad is seen first), system reconstruction, psychodrama, guided fantasy, system sculpting, therapist as communications model/teacher.	Focuses on behavior and communication patterns; one therapist, with one or more therapists behind a one-way mirror; straightforward advice, directives, and so on, with compliant families; paradoxical interventions with non-compliant families.	

Name of Founder / Name of Therapy	Salvador Minuchin Structural Therapy	Carl Whitaker Symbolic/Experiential Therapy	
View of system	A system is more than the individual biopsychodynamics of its members. System members relate according to certain arrangements that govern their transactions. These	The system is an integrated whole, and each member derives the freedom to individuate and separate from the system through a sense of belonging to the whole.	

(Continued)

	arrangements form a whole: the structure of the system.	The power of the system—for good or for ill—is the key to individual growth and development.
The healthy system	The well-functioning system has an underlying organizational structure that allows for fluid and flexible responses to changing conditions through the system life cycle. Thus, the system provides both for mutual support and for the autonomy of its individual members.	Health is a process of perceptual becoming. The healthy system: has a sense of wholeness, maintains generational boundaries along with role flexibility, is creative and playful, encourages the expression of autonomy, and grows despite adversity and resultant stress.
Dysfunction	Symptoms arise when system structures are inflexible, whether enmeshed or disengaged, and the system does not make appropriate structural adjustments; the system responds in an inflexible manner to changing conditions in the system life cycle.	Dysfunctional systems are characterized by interactional rigidity and emotional deadness. The specific symptom is often related to the pre-established roles and triangles of system members. Symptoms serve to maintain the status quo.
Role of therapist	The therapist's role is paradoxical: supportive while challenging, attacking while encouraging, being for the system yet *against* the dysfunctional system. The therapist is an active, authoritative agent of	The therapist focuses on *being* full of the client/system; to use him/herself to help system members fully express/communicate what they are experiencing. The therapist is highly active but usually not very

Table 1.1 (Continued)

Name of Founder / Name of Therapy	Murray Bowen / Multigenerational Therapy	James Framo / Object-Relations Therapy	Ivan Boszormnenyi-Nagy / Contextual Therapy
	change: an actor, director, and producer in system change.	directive—a coach or a surrogate grandparent; co-therapy is normative.	
Goal of therapy	The basic goal is the restructuring of the system's system of transactional rules, such that interactions become more flexible, with expanded availability of alternative ways for system members to relate to one another.	The goal is growth and creativity rather than reduction of symptoms because individual growth and creative freedom will reduce the need for the symptom; growth occurs when system members are able to experience the present moment and communicate that experience with other system members.	
Primary techniques	Structural/system mapping: "joining" techniques: maintenance, tracking, accommodation, mimesis; "disequilibrating" techniques: reframing, use of metaphors, enactment, boundary marking, blocking, punctuation, unbalancing.	The therapist as a person as a primary technique; conjoint therapy and the use of a co-therapist is the norm; reframing; modeling; therapeutic absurdity; affective confrontation; fantasy; paradoxical intentions; "as if" situations.	

the most practiced and researched forms of couples counseling in the most recent phase. While a lot continues to occur in the field, there is not much that is additive to the story of the development of TCC, so we will leave the history lesson and pivot to how the development of couples counseling intersects with the idea of TCC.

How History Points the Way to Tandem Couples Counseling

The treatment of couples has experienced impressive growth. From its beginnings as a form of individual-focused prevention modality to the early psychoanalysts willing to push the boundaries of their theory to include relationship dynamics within the analysis, and later to see the couple together, to the development of seeing the couple and family as an integrated system, larger than the individual units, the field has rapidly evolved in less than 100 years. Such a dynamic field encourages innovation. Just like those early pioneers, the expansiveness of relationships calls us to look for new ways of helping couples. TCC draws upon this history and provides an innovative pathway to ameliorating relationship dysfunction.

As couples counseling evolved and systems theory took shape, conjoint meetings became the norm, if not the standard for treating the couple. If we asked you to picture "couples counseling," you would conjure an image of one counselor, in a comfortable chair, sitting across from a couple on a couch. But what became of those early innovations such as concurrent, collaborative, and combined collaborative ways of working with the couple? The short answer is they all but disappeared from the research literature, replaced solely by that image of one counselor, two clients.

Concurrent therapy is found in few places in literature and during our numerous training on TCC, we would invariably be approached during the break by an attendee who would report they were "doing essentially the same thing" as TCC in their current practice. As we discussed the particulars of said "thing," we uncovered substantial differences. In all cases, the therapists were talking about concurrent treatment—where they, or someone they know, routinely see the couple for a few individual sessions. Of the reasons given for meeting individually with couples, the most common were:

The need to gather background information.

2 The conflict was too high during conjoint sessions, so the individual meetings provided a way to continue the treatment but in a less intense environment.

3 The progress had become stagnant and individual counseling became a way to break through the impasse.

4 One of the clients requested it.

All the potential rationales for including individuals in couples counseling make sense, but a scant amount of literature is cautious with the shift from purely conjoint to concurrent. There seems to exist an inherent distrust of individual counseling with couples; part of this schism might exist due to the interwoven histories of marital and family counseling. As Olson (1970) noted, "Whereas both fields began to develop at the same time historically, the reason for their development came from quite different sources. Marital therapy grew out of the social need for practitioners to deal with marital problems, while family therapists began their practice because they increasingly realized the inadequacy of exclusively using individual treatment techniques with their clients" (p. 505). While marital counseling routinely utilized concurrent treatment, the faith in individual counseling diminished as it began to merge with family counseling. We postulate that this primarily comes from a philosophical incongruence between the dominant Systems Theory and the modality of individual counseling that is inherent in the history of the profession and rooted in the theory. This distrust is unfortunate, given the fact research suggests individual sessions can produce positive outcomes in couples in certain situations (Gurman & Burton, 2014).

While the reasons for concurrent treatment listed above are singularly clinical rationales, clients may request individual sessions based on intrapersonal motives. Beck (1989) writes about this use of concurrent therapy as potentially problematic:

A cautious approach to the use of concurrent individual sessions in marital treatment is necessary because of the complex nature of marital relationships. Concurrent treatment of couples is defined as a process in which each spouse is seen in individual sessions by the same therapist. One partner often expresses a desire to have the therapist to himself to gain an ally (Beck, 1989), to share a secret

(Martin and Bird, 1963) or to seek relief from some inner turmoil (Zinner, 1976). Acceding to such a request can lead to unwanted outcomes if careful consideration of its implication is not given for each partner, the course of treatment, or the marriage in general. The other partner may experience a sense of abandonment or a fear that he or she will not be heard or understood. Granting an individual interview may imply that the marital issues are secondary and will subtly reinforce further distance (p. 231).

Overall, the use of individual counseling as a part of the couple's treatment has been both a regularly employed yet distrusted modality. Purists of Systems Theory will resist the possible benefits of individual counseling, while clinicians will often use individual sessions when stuck. While it is safe to say that the use of individual sessions in couples counseling is an often utilized ed strategy by practitioners, the reasons are not well studied or consistently applied. We were intrigued by the role of the individual sessions as we approached our work with couples, and we will explore more of this later.

As for other innovations of collaborative and combined collaborative treatments, they fared less well in the literature, and how prevalent they are in actual practice is undetermined. We had questions about the utility of using some of the elements of these approaches. From history, we pulled the following pieces for further exploration:

1 Use of concurrent individual sessions
2 Assignation of one counselor for each client
3 Implementation of conjoint sessions as a foursome
4 Utilization of counselor consultation

These elements became the foundation for TCC but moving the ideas into practice with a cohesive structure would take more time. The next section returns to where we began in this chapter, with our historical experiences that lead to the formation of TCC.

The Evolution of TCC

Traditional couples counseling is effective for large numbers of couples— we make no criticism of the status of the couple's treatment. At the same time, we recognize that counseling is a human endeavor so structural and philosophical challenges that require useful alternatives will always exist. In the sections that follow, we illustrate some of these problems we grappled with as clinicians and we offer what we consider to be serviceable methods for overcoming them. These ideas help form the foundation of TCC.

Structural Problems

Couple's counseling is offered most consistently in office settings where a couple (two clients) interact with a counselor. The triad structure has been the standard for decades and it is no surprise that it is the most widely used format today. Counselors, depending on theoretical orientation, interact with the couple to help them overcome individual problems or problems between them by focusing on relationship issues. Each focus has merits and clients benefit from efforts to help them individually or interpersonally.

Concerns about the structural problems surfaced when we began receiving several referrals from other counselors. These counselors often referred couples to us because they were either concerned about the lack of progress or they were treating an individual who wanted to remain in individual counseling but needed a referral for couples counseling. Word had gotten out to the professional community that we were developing a new protocol for couples' work and that it might be of help to partners who had tried traditional couples counseling without success. Because of these referrals, our intake process included an expanded range of questions about previous therapies. We asked new clients to provide detailed assessments of what helped and hindered their progress in the earlier therapies. The clients' honesty impressed us; they easily recalled the helpful moments, the stressful moments, their reasons for terminating, and how sessions affected the quality of their relationships. They were very respectful of their previous providers and believed their counselors were doing the best they could. To us, this seemed a bit odd, given that some of these couples endured some very trying times and obtained little relief during their couples' counseling sessions. This anomaly became the first clue to what may be structurally problematic. It was during one intake interview that a client shared the following story. He said:

The sessions became tough for both of us. One week my wife would get the focus on her problems. The next week it would be my turn. Frankly, I would be relieved when it was her week, but I still did not like seeing her upset during the session and for a few days after. I'm not sure if she felt the same way about me when it was my week to get criticized.

Now, a perceptive reader might respond to this client's experience by saying, "That is just bad couples counseling! The counselor was doing individual counseling in a couple's session and failed to focus on the mutuality of the relationship." This assertion would be correct if this were the end of the story, but it speaks to a larger structural problem with traditional couples counseling: traditional couples counseling creates an inherent triangle that is difficult to manage, depending on the severity and intensity of the couple dynamics. Within this triangle, it is not only difficult for the counselor to maintain balance, but it is exceedingly difficult for the clients to feel that the counselor is not "taking sides."

This "side taking" perception is damaging to the clients and produces feelings of blame, shame, and can manifest in a wide variety of re- sistance strategies—all of which damage the therapeutic momentum. Within this dynamic, clients conclude that there was one "bad" person who needed repair in the couple, and one healthy person. It is perceived that the role shifted and was determined by the counselor, as evidenced by who the counselor sided with at any given time.

We knew some of the counselors the couples had seen and were suspicious about the client's conclusions, so we asked how they knew the side taking was occurring. To our surprise, they relied entirely upon whom the counselor attended. They perceived counselor eye contact as affirmation and the lack thereof as condemnation or deduction. We realized that with three people in the room, the counselor was always focusing on one or the other client and that attention was immediately—correctly or incorrectly—interpreted by the clients. The structural problem was simple: one counselor can only focus on one person at a time and who the counselor focuses on is as important as who the counselor "ignores." At this point, the clients' proper com- plaint about "counselor side-taking" had two easily identified elements. One, the counselors would inadvertently validate one client more than the other, depending on the issue, and his judgment about who might be "right" and "wrong." And two, the simple fact that counselors can only attend to one person at a time had an enormous impact on how the clients perceived what the attention meant. This analysis became the first clue that having two counselors in the same room with a couple might have immense structural benefits. There is no possibility of being attended to if the counselor is attending to your partner in a traditional setting.

As we will discuss more in-depth in later chapters, there is always the possibility of being attended to by a counselor while your partner is being attended to by another counselor in TCC. While on its surface it may not sound too important, clients with histories and complicated relationship problems are especially sensitive to situations where they feel unheard and any competition for attention exists. Sadly, how these clients each perceived the relationship between their partner and the counselor could have profound negative impacts upon the session and on their relationship—the very thing they were trying to heal. The situation could best be termed an iatrogenic effect—a provider-induced problem or a worsening of the already problematic conditions. While no couple's counselor would intentionally worsen the symptoms they were trying to treat, a structural problem in the delivery of those services could inadvertently produce such unwanted outcomes.

The process of interviewing clients who experienced earlier problematic couple's therapies further illuminated the overwhelmingly complicated concern of side-taking, while providing services to struggling couples. Our training in systems theory made us uniquely sensitive to triangulation and the threats to intimacy that triangulation can produce. The reality of traditional couples counseling—three people in the counseling office—raises important questions about how a single triangle will affect the clinical process. The answer is a simple, yet worrisome, truth: every single interaction between the counselor and one client is a triangulation where one client is in and the other is out. The effect may be severe or subtle, but it will always be present. When a client claims that the counselor always takes up for their partner and decides to quit therapy because he or she feels "scapegoated," we can see the intense reaction to the triangulation, while more subtle responses include resistance to fully invest in the process, reluctance to explore new modes of relating, or quiet attempts to sabotage the effort.

Given the known structural problems with traditional approaches to couples counseling, we believe that TCC offers serviceable structural alternatives that limit the negative effects of triangulation, especially for couples who have histories of complicated relationship issues and poor models for intimacy. TCC also seeks to improve outcomes by urging the clients to think in terms of the relationship instead of themselves. Stressing a focus on the relationship makes it much easier for couples to assess their collective strengths and weaknesses and develop strategies for improving in an environment that reduces defensiveness, shame, and resentment in both clients. In other words, TCC changes both the structure of the therapy setting (two counselors and two clients) and the focus. TCC is a response to two structural or strategic goals: (1) reduce or eliminate adverse effects of triangulation and (2) avoid the prevalent possibility of "side-taking" by focusing on the relationship instead of the individuals. How these goals are accomplished, why this alternative protocol works, and for whom it works best will all be covered in the remainder of the text.

The Role of Fear and Balancing the Issue of Individual Needs and the Relationship

Working with a range of clients and being able to see them in TCC sessions provided fertile territory for us to develop alternative ideas about the cause of struggles within couples. Our discussions sought to understand why couples tend to not improve and hypothesize about the conditions that seem immutable within the relationship. Eventually, we concluded that there often existed an overarching feeling shared by both partners—one that was never openly expressed to one another. We saw plenty of anger and frustration focused on topics that warranted less intense reactions. These observations caused us to conclude that there had to be an underlying feeling responsible for most of the strife within the couple. Consulting literature and each other, we identified anger as the emotion of greatest concern to the couple, so in our early work, we frequently helped clients explore the underlying concerns that propelled their anger but most of the other interventions we employed usually fall short in our evaluation. Over time, it became clear to us that the feeling was not anger—it was fear.—and in all cases, it was fear of intimacy.

That's not to say that the anger was irrelevant, it's just that when someone is afraid it becomes impossible to safely share information with the perceived source of threat and the situation can be crippling.

Intimacy is often associated with physical intimacy in Western Culture that when the topic was first introduced to clients, they agreed—assuming we were talking about sex when we meant emotional, spiritual, and social intimacy. We let clients know that there is a way of communicating with one another that had profound, positive possibilities. However, it could be a source of great fear as it requires them to be vulnerable to a person who knows them so well and could hurt them deeply; it was a double-edged sword. We also knew that many of the couples had observed families where fear of intimacy was rampant. They had been "trained" to manage that fear by being angry, controlling, dismissive, sarcastic, and even physically abusive. Fear had a profound negative impact on these couples who, despite their struggles, were still searching for a functional way of obtaining the fruits of their relationships.

These fear-based reactions were not confined to the client's relationship. As counselors, we knew that we could easily become the subject of their anger. They might have secrets they were afraid we would somehow expose; they might fear being judged, or they might sense that we would blame one of them for *all* the problems of the couple. We knew we were experienced enough to manage from our end, but we also knew that they could react angrily once they perceive us as threatening despite our efforts. It would take a good deal of time for us to finally settle upon the overarching source of their fear—the propellant for their anger—and eventually the overarching focus of our TCC clinical work.

We also reasoned that to be successful we would need to change the focus from the individuals in the relationship to the Relationship. We had seen so many sessions where clients arrived with the rigid expectation that couples counseling was a place where you get *your* needs met. Client complaints were always focused on the partner and their inability or unwillingness to give the other what they needed. This tug-of-war went nowhere and entertaining it was a perilous journey. We had to replace the individual neediness with something larger than either of the two people. The Battle Royale over whose needs would get met first only put counselors in one unjustified position after another. It also fueled triangulation concerns into raging fires. In a society where individual needs reign supreme, this would be no easy task.

Our discussions headed toward the idea of making the relationship more important than either of the people's individual needs. We surmised that this was a reasonable re-focus but because of its potential to create more fear in the couple, it would have to be done very carefully and deliberately. We thought it would be a difficult idea for the couple to grasp; however, we were quickly proven wrong. Upon sharing the idea about the overarching importance of the relationship focus and not the individuals, it calmed the conflict and brought some relief to the couple; they seemed to know that the way they were thinking about each other was making things worse and it might help to try a different approach. We often use this metaphor to help explain our suggestion: when you first learn to hit a baseball with a bat, you tend to look at the bat and not the ball and the result is that you never hit the ball. When the coach finally asks you to hold the bat and keep your eyes on the ball, the new batter is shocked and happily surprised as the ball sails off the end of the bat.

The exclusive focus on the relationship was an enormous boon for us. When one or another member of the couple would "act out," our comments were predictable and surprisingly useful to the couple. We would simply ask: did your behavior help the relationship, hurt the relationship, or keep it about the same? Shaming comments, siding with one or the other member of the couple, judging of all kinds had now been reduced to a choice between three options: better, worse, or about the same. Clients became so used to the routine that they would sit down for their session, and without any prompting, simply announce that their actions affected the relationship this week, in this way. The family of origin issues that so heavily influenced the couple would now have a safer environment to be discussed and worked through.

The focus on the relationship also provided a pathway for avoiding scapegoating and blaming. We recognized that if a person is perceived to be responsible for another's pain, the likelihood to talk about what they had done or try to do to repair the injury, is low. If they are not solely to blame, restoration and healing are much more likely to occur. It was abundantly clear to us that a couple was really an amalgam of family of origin issues—some are adaptive, and some are not—but all affecting the life of the couple. If we dealt with the individuals all we would have are individuals who knew about their "issues." By focusing on the couple, we were now dealing with the stage the issues played out their roles in. In real-time we could enter the stage as a pair of therapists using our relationship to help heal their relationship. This point became increasingly important because it was finally obvious: the counselor's relationship could be effectively used to heal the couple's relationship. And so TCC began as an alternative focus and protocol to helping couples develop the type of relationship that any two people fortunate enough to find each other should have.

Creating an Environment of Empathy and Listening

Our work also revealed that clients had poor methods for noticing what was happening within their partners. Fear made understanding the other's emotional, spiritual, and intimacy needs exceedingly difficult, even risky. This reality became a source of concern because it had to be safely overcome, or the fears of intimacy would continue to wreck the relationships in ways that could make it irreparable. We concluded that the clients would need a tool to help them overcome fear and improve intimacy levels and that tool came in the form of "Compassionate Listening" drawn from Buddhist teachings. This is a method of listening deeply to a person that can only be used in only one circumstance; for the Buddhists, Compassionate Listening is used solely to ease suffering in another human being. We agreed that most of our clients were suffering from a range of family of origin experiences but were too afraid, for exceptionally good reasons, to allow anyone in close enough to help them hear. The focus on the couple's relationship could now include the idea that one's partner could be a source of healing once the level of fear is controlled, and then the couple could find sensible ways of sharing their suffering, in place of conflict, with one another. The most important purpose of the couple's relationships is to help the individuals heal from the pains and injuries they sustained at an earlier time in their lives. Through compassionate listening, couples could heal one another and, in the process, create a loving and supportive environment to live—raise children if they wished—and relate effectively to others.

We believe that clients want their couple relationships to be helpful to one another and they want it to exist as a shelter from the pain, uncertainty, and sadness inhabiting the world. When couples understand that it is within their power to create such an environment and learn methods to help each other and their families, they tend to buy into the process. We would often ask couples if they had any training, experience, or direction in establishing and maintaining a healthy family environment, most of them said no. While they knew that they had trouble creating what they wanted they kept doing what they see from others; however, their models were problematic, and following them was counterproductive.

Couples, we learned, have corners that form retreat zones where they each head to once anxiety builds or fear inhabits their daily lives. For example, when a couple experiences financial distress, one member of the couples might isolate while the other member might begin to nag. Ironically, the increase in one's cornering behavior also increases the other's. The result is an easily identifiable nagging-retreating response, which anyone who has ever done couples counseling could relate to—as the other retreats the angrier the nagger gets; the more the nagger nags, the angrier the retreater becomes. The problem here is that there is no practical way to resolve the anger because anger is not the issue. The problem is fear and the role it plays in each of the couple's family of origin. By directing the couple to honor the fear and deal with each other by listening compassionately, one not only begins to resolve the pain derived from the family but also begins to solve the financial problem burdening the couple.

The idea of anger and fear relative to the family also had intriguing applications for creating a more compassionate couple's environment. We often encountered reactions from one of the couples towards their partner that defied reasonable explanation; one of the couples might be incredulous and emotionally inconsolable about an event that seemingly does not warrant that level of emotion. Asking the clients about the "overreaction" tends to intensify the reaction. Since we were identifying so many rich patterns in each member's family history, it seemed reasonable to assume that the explanation for the intensity existed in the past.

We decided to begin a process where we ask the "overly upset" clients in one or another situation if they could assign a percentage to the source of their distress. In other words, we ask, "What percent of your anger is directly attributable to your partner's behavior, and what—if applicable—percent has happened to you in the past?" At first, clients reacted negatively and become sarcastic or upset about not being understood properly, and even react angrily towards either or both of us. They perceived the question as siding with their partner and downplaying their internal pain. After taking some time to carefully explain the reason for our question, clients would venture into the possibility that their anger could have more than one source. As the clients became more comfortable with this idea, they began to hypothesize about alternate sources of their pain and frustration. The result was quite interesting and eminently useful. Many partners would apologize easier for their mistakes if they knew that they were taking part of the responsibility, while the rest could be placed on their partner's earlier life experiences.

Remarkably, some partners were able to employ Compassionate Listening skills when their significant other began talking about the sadness and frustration they had sustained earlier in their lives. This alternative gave clients a first-hand experience at helping one another heal, even if they were partially responsible for the pain their partner experienced. Once a client realizes how much pain their partner had endured over something they had done, they were less likely to do it again. We commonly heard comments like, "if I had known how severely injured he was being so harshly criticized by his father, I would have NEVER said what I just said to him," "I love him and had no idea that history even existed," "I hope there is something I could do to help him feel better about being treated so harshly," and finally, "my mother was my harshest critic and she was relentless. Maybe my experiences with a similar problem could be of help to him."

Conclusion

We hope the brief exploration of the history of couples counseling and how it intersects with our emerging ideas about TCC provided a useful foundation to frame the remainder of the text. The primary takeaway is that the TCC approach was created out of clinical curiosity and client needs, much like the early experimentation with concurrent and conjoint counseling one hundred years ago. It is important to note that presenting an alternative to traditional couples counseling is not saying that other forms of couples counseling are universally ineffective. In fact, research shows that couples counseling has a positive impact on a wide variety of mental health issues. Stratton et al. (2015) conducted a meta-analysis of all couple related outcome studies in the years between 2000 and 2009 and found promising and consistent positive outcomes of couples counseling for a wide variety of presenting problems and populations. There also exists a compelling amount of research on specific theoretical approaches and populations that substantiates the effectiveness of traditional forms of couples counseling (Ahmadi, Rasouli, Alaf, & Zadi, 2014; Denton, Wittenborn, & Golden, 2012; Rathgeber et al., 2019; Shadish & Baldwin, 2005; Von Sydow, Beher, Schweitzer, & Retzlaff, 2010).

What we are offering is meant to be an addition to other forms of couples counseling. It is a synthesis of practices from individual, couples, and group counseling designed to address high conflict stagnation in relational dysfunction. It is within the combination of these traditions that make the application of TCC unique from other forms of counseling. Counseling, in general, and couples counseling, in particular, are rapidly evolving fields and our contribution in this text exists as but one small step in a much larger effort that continuously seeks greater levels of effectiveness and improved options for the masses who struggle with interpersonal, psychological, societal, and career or vocational challenges.

The following chapters offer theoretical foundations for the model, philosophical pillars upon which some of the approaches are based, examples on how the therapy can be conducted, alternative populations that have been successfully helped, and methods and techniques for consultation and supervision of the TCC counselors. We are delighted to bring you along on this journey of discovery and hope that the remaining chapters will provide sufficient information that allows you, in consort with a co-counselor, to explore the benefits of TCC.

References

Ahmadi, M., Rasouli, M., Alaf, C. B., & Zadi, F. S. (2014). Effectiveness of emotion-focused couple therapy in marital commitment and emotion regulation. *International Journal of Psychology and Behavioral Research. Special Issue, 1*(1), 54–63.

Beck, R. L. (1989). The individual interview in couples treatment. *Journal of Family Therapy, 11,* 231–241.

Capuzzi, D., & Stauffer, M. D. (2015). *Foundations of couples, marriage, and family counseling.* New York: Wiley.

Denton, W. H., Wittenborn, A. K., & Golden, R. N. (2012). Augmenting antidepressant medication treatment of depressed women with emotionally focused therapy for couples: A randomized pilot study. *Journal of Marital and Family Therapy, 38,* 23–38.

Kerr, M. E., & Bowen, M. (1988). *Family evaluation: An approach based on Bowen theory.* New York: Norton.

Gladding, S. (2018). *Family therapy: History, theory, and practice* (7th ed.). New York: Merrill.

Gottman, J. M. (1994). *Why marriages succeed or fail.* New York: Simon and Schuster.

Gottman, J. M. (1999). *The marriage clinic: A scientifically based marital therapy.* New York: Norton.

Greene, B., & Solomon, A. (1963). Marital disharmony: Concurrent psychoanalytic therapy of husband and wife by the same psychiatrist. *American Journal of Psychiatry, 17,* 443–450.

Gurman, A. S., & Burton, M. (2014). Individual therapy for couple problems: Perspectives and pitfalls. *Journal of Marital and Family Therapy, 40*(4), 470–483.

Gurman, A. S., & Fraenkel, P. (2002). The history of couple therapy: A millennial review. *Family Process, 41*(2), 199–260.

Gurman, A. S., Lebow, J. L., & Snyder, D. K. (2015). *Clinical handbook of couple therapy* (5th ed.). New York: Guilford Press.

Johnson, S. (1996). *The practice of emotionally focused marital therapy.* New York: Brunner Mazel.

Martin, P, & Bird, W. (1963). An approach to psychotherapy of marriage partners: The stereoscopic technique. *Psychiatry, 16,* 123–127.

Mittelman, B. (1948). The concurrent analysis of marital couples. *Psychoanalytic Quarterly, 17,* 182–197.

Olson, D. H. (1970). Marital and family therapy: Integrative review and critique. *Journal of Marriage and the Family, 32*(4), 501–538.

Paterson, J., (2009). Looking in the Mirror. Counseling Today. https://ct. counseling.org/2009/05/looking-in-the-mirror/.

Prochaska, J., & Prochaska, J. (1978). Twentieth century trends in marriage and marital therapy. In T. J. Paolino & B. S. McCrady (Eds), *Marriage and Marital Therapy* (pp. 1–24). New York: Brunner Mazel.

Rathgeber, M., Bürkner, P., Schiller, E., Holling, H., Bürkner, P. C., & Schiller, E.-M. (2019). The efficacy of emotionally focused couples therapy and behavioral couples therapy: A meta-analysis. *Journal of Marital & Family Therapy, 45*(3), 447–463.

Royce, J., & Hogan, P. (1960). *Co-therapy in a special situation.* Paper delivered at the American Group Psychotherapy Association.

Sager, C J. (1967). The conjoint session in marriage therapy. *The American Journal of Psychoanalysis, 27*(1), 139–146.

Shadish, W. R., & Baldwin, S. A. (2005). Effects of behavioral marital therapy: A meta-analysis of randomized controlled trials. *Journal of Consulting and Clinical Psychology, 73*(1), 6–14.

Stratton, P., Silver, E., Nascimento, N., McDonnell, L., Powell, G., & Nowotny, E. (2015). Couple and family therapy outcome research in the previous decade: What does the evidence tell us? *Contemporary Family Therapy: An International Journal, 37*(1), 1–12.

Stuart, R. B. (1980). *Helping couples change: A social learning approach to marital therapy.* New York: Guilford.

Von Sydow, K., Beher, S., Schweitzer, J., & Retzlaff, R. (2010). The efficacy of systemic therapy with adult patients: A meta-content analysis of 38 randomized controlled trials. *Family Process, 49*(4), 457–485.

2

DEFINING AND ASSESSING HIGH CONFLICT COUPLES

It will come as no surprise that conflict—and how to mediate it—has been at the core of the couple's therapy since its establishment. Heitler (1990) defines conflict as, "a situation in which seemingly incompatible elements exert force in opposing or divergent directions" (p. 5). While conflict is normal in every relationship, high conflict connotes a level that exceeds one's expectations, and what could be considered as healthy for the relationship. While normal levels of conflict can be productive for relational growth, elevated levels of conflict can impede growth potential for the relationship. This notion of "high conflict couples" and the impact of treatment has been a topic of discussion and exploration for decades (Cohen & Levite, 2012; Fraenkel, 2019; Friedman, 2004; Gottman, 1993; Gottman & Silver, 1999). What we see when we look at literature and our own clinical experience is a continuum of conflict intensity that often reaches a point where treatment fails, and the couple gets locked into a cycle of pain. It is these dynamics that we are exploring with the work of Tandem Couples Counseling (TCC).

It is important to note that when we use the term "high conflict couple," we are not assessing equal responsibility or blame for the conflict. The term "high conflict" is meant as a descriptive term—one that illuminates the intensity of the conflict within the couple. While it is assumed that each person in the relationship has some role to play in the relationship dynamics, these roles are will be identified as the counseling unfolds. It is interesting that it is often the intensity of the conflict characterizing these relationships that so often interferes with the exploration and rapport-building phase of traditional couples' work.

High conflict is highlighted here because the elements of high conflict couples can contribute to treatment failure or stagnation, which opens the door for a possible TCC intervention. Anderson, Anderson, Palmer, Mutchler, and Baker (2011) asserted that the field did not offer a clear distinction of what constitutes a high conflict and concluded that this lack of clarity produces little basis or direction for intervention within this population. Because the experience of high conflict couples can lead to TCC, we thought it important to explore and define the concepts of a high conflict couple before we introduce the details of the treatment protocol.

Defining High Conflict in Couples

Typologies: Two Models

Gottman (1993) outlined what is the most cited high conflict typologies as part of the overall typology structure he uses for assessing potential success or failure in relationships. Within his approach, he identifies five couple types, with three (volatile, hostile, and hostile/detached) being considered a high conflict. Volatile couples are considered by Gottman to be a stable couple type and are differentiated from the other two types by a higher quantity of positive statements about the marriage. However, the high frequency of tension, defensiveness, and conflict are also inherent in the volatile type. Hostile and hostile/detached are labeled unstable by Gottman, as they are most likely to result in relationship termination. Hostile and hostile/detached are differentiated by the general approach to conflict—engaged or avoidant. Hostile couples are engaged in persistent negative interactions, full of contempt and defensiveness, while hostile/detached use withdrawal and avoidance to slowly suffocate the relationship.

Gottman and Silver (1999) adds the "Four Horsemen of the Apocalypse" (p. 27) to the illustration of elements that contribute to conflict and divorce. These destructive dynamics include criticism, contempt, defensiveness, and stonewalling. Each will be discussed below as they are important in identifying high conflict couples.

Criticism: It is normal to be dissatisfied in relationships. The issue, however, is not the dissatisfaction but how that dissatisfaction is conveyed within the couple. According to Gottman and Silver (1999), criticism can be distinguished from a complaint by the focus of the statement. Complaints are issue-focused, while criticism is personal and therefore more damaging. For example, saying "I wish you wouldn't say terrible things about my mom. I feel defensive when you do that" (complaint) is different from "You have no right to say that about my mom. You are a mean, ungrateful, jealous man!" (criticism). When focusing on behavior, a complaint decreases the attack and increases the likelihood of change. The criticism is destructive because it distracts from the needed behavior change by emphasizing the personal attack. The purpose of criticism is to wound and hurt the other person.

Contempt: This element of high conflict arises from the feeling that your partner and their needs are not worthy of time or consideration. It conveys an element of disgust that is demeaning to the other person. Contempt typically manifests in sarcasm, anger, eye-rolling, and hurtful jokes.

Denise: There are plenty of times I try to help, but you don't seem to notice.

Fred: Oh, yeah? What is it you do actually?

Denise: I do a lot. I don't feel like making an itemized list for you.

Fred: That's because you can't. I mean, come on, name one thing of value you did yesterday while I was at work?

Denise: I made 20 gift bags for the church volunteer luncheon.

Fred: Oh, Jesus Christ, my mistake. I'm sorry, I did not acknowledge that huge contribution to the family you did there. Please, take the rest of the week off.

Defensiveness: Defensiveness in high conflict couples can appear in two harmful ways. Gottman focuses on defensiveness as a natural outgrowth of an attacking and contemptuous relationship. In this arrangement, one partner goes on the attack, and the other moves into a defense mode. Partners can switch roles, but the outcome is always the same: no healthy resolution. In the following interaction, you can almost feel Mark crawling deeper into his shell as Kitty tries to draw him out.

Kitty: I just don't understand why you can't initiate fun stuff for us to do.

Mark: I mean, I do, sometimes.

Kitty: I don't even know what that means. The issue is you don't do it and you don't make me a priority. You are either lazy or don't care about me.

Mark: I think I do care.

Kitty: How? Do you really think you show me even the slightest bit of attention? Everything we do, I have to plan. If you had it your way, we would sit in the house and watch TV, probably in different rooms, every single day. How is that a relationship?

Mark: That's not true.

Kitty: How can you say that? I bet you can't name one thing you planned in the past month. Don't even try. You'll just embarrass yourself. That's all I need right now ... you feeling embarrassed. If that happens, he won't talk for a week.

Mark: (Silence)

Fall and Howard (2017) also highlighted how the defenses of minimization, denial, and blame can also be used to avoid responsibility in a relationship. Minimization deflates the impact of the behavior to decrease the intensity of the consequence. "I only cheated on her once." Denial attempts to avoid the consequence altogether by saying the behavior never occurred, even when there is ample evidence of the behavior. "I never cheated on her. Those texts are from someone else. I don't know how they got on my phone." Blame is the most destructive, as it tries to move the consequence away from the person who chose the behavior and onto another person, usually the receiver of the behavior. "I cheated because you weren't paying any attention to me. If you would have been a better wife, this would have never happened."

Stonewalling: Stonewalling is active behavioral and emotional disengagement from the relationship. It is much more intense than defensiveness because in most cases, the person completely disconnects from the conversation, leaving the partner frustrated and helpless—like trying to get a turtle out of its shell. If the turtle doesn't want to come out, there is no way to get it out without destroying the shell or the turtle. Stonewalling stagnates the change process. The stonewaller feels isolated, yet safe, behind the wall. This isolation cuts the person off from the relationship and any growth. The person on the other side of the wall has two options: walk away and participate in the avoidance or set siege to the stonewall, but either tactic is not healthy for the relationship.

> George: This happens every time we have a discussion. You just clam up.
>
> Martha: I don't know.
>
> George: Well, talk about how you feel about the disagreement we had this weekend. I mean, your solution was to just walk away and avoid me all weekend. Now we are here in counseling and you can't run. We need to address it.
>
> Martha: (shrugs) I don't know what you want me to say.
>
> George: I want you to tell me why you allowed our son to go on the sailing trip without talking to me first like we agreed.
>
> Martha: (shrugs)
>
> George: You know what? Forget it. Two can play that game. We'll just sit here and stare at the counselor and make her figure it out.

Anderson et al. (2011) proposed another well thought out and grounded model of high conflict typologies. In their model, high conflict can be defined by two clusters. "Cluster I: Pervasive Negative Exchanges is characterized by recurring destructive communication patterns, defensiveness and counterattacking, rapid escalation of the conflict, unremitting change attempts, continual rejections of such attempts, and negative attributions. Cluster II: Hostile, Insecure Emotional Environment is characterized by strong negative affect, a lack of safety, a sense of mutual distrust, emotional reactivity, triangulation, and enmeshment" (p. 16). It was their assertion that the clusters and the behaviors—thought and feelings therein—would produce high levels of stable and intense conflict that would produce frequent negative treatment outcomes.

For Cluster I: Pervasive Negative exchanges, the high conflict couple's patterns are distinguished by persistent interactions "characterized by defensiveness, aggression, and shared and rigid portrayals of the other" (Anderson et al., 2011, p. 16). The communication between the members of the couple is conflict based. Any conversation, no matter how seemingly light and innocuous, often erupts into an intense battle. Within these exchanges, each member will often adopt an extremely defensive position. The defensive strategies can include avoidance, blame, denial, withdrawal, and efforts to control the behavior of the partner. Cohen, Luxenburg, Dattner, and Martz (1999) noted that the elevated level of defensive behavior of high conflict couples made mediation much more challenging.

Counselor:	So you both wrote, "Communication skills" on the intake form as something you wanted to work on in counseling.
Julie:	Yes, he can't talk to me without yelling, so that would be something to change.
Counselor:	I can see how yelling could negatively impact a conversation. What would you like to change about your communication style?
Julie:	I would like him to stop being such a prick all the time. Does that count?
Frank:	Oh, look! Little Miss Perfect over here (laughs).

Julie:	See, that's what I'm talking about. Prick sarcastic behavior. This is why we fight. You can't handle criticism and your mom didn't teach you to respect women.
Counselor:	Let's stick to communication for a minute...
Julie (yelling):	I'm talking about communication, but no one will listen to me!
Frank:	Honestly, I don't know what she's talking about, so I'll just sit here and listen until you (counselor) calm her down.
Julie (still yelling):	Don't you do that, you scumbag. You're not going to sit there, all smug, and pretend to not know what is going on. This is why your last wife cheated on you with your brother.
Frank:	(gets on his phone)

Along with the quality and consistency of the intense and defensive behavior common in high conflict couples, there is also an increase in aggressive content. The aggression is distinguished from non-high conflict couples in its tendency to be person-focused, rather than issue-focused. High conflict couples tend to personalize issues, so the attacks are personal as well. It is important to note that the aggression seems to differ from domestic violence in that it is more mutual and less dominated by power and control dynamics. However, it is important for counselors to assess the presence of physical and sexual abuse, as that will impact your treatment trajectory. We will address domestic violence later in the chapter, so for now, the escalating personal attacks are illustrated below.

Counselor:	Tell me more about the decision making about the vacation.
Eric:	What decision making? She's a control freak and must have everything her way or no way.
Sue:	I'm a control freak? What about dinner last night? You are such a weakling; you couldn't even decide what to eat. Grow a spine, you piece of shit.

> Counselor: So, moving back to the decision-making process about the vacation...

Lastly, high conflict couples possess and utilize rigidly held negative beliefs about the other partner. These beliefs color every interaction and behavior within the couple and make change very difficult because regardless of the behavior or the intent, the other partner will attribute evil intent and behave as if some transgression has occurred against them. Beliefs of "he is deliberately trying to hurt me" or "she is willingly denying me happiness" are common core beliefs that we have seen in high conflict couples over the years. As one can imagine, having this extremely negative belief system filter every interaction makes traditional couples work challenging, as it is virtually impossible to define a mutual goal.

> Counselor: As you considered coming to counseling, what is the one hope you had about the process of counseling and its impact on your relationship?
>
> Luis: I'm not sure she really wants to change. That's my fear.
>
> Counselor: That's a fear. What about hope?
>
> Luis: I mean, I just think she wants to make my life miserable. She does things that she knows will drive me crazy and she does them anyway just to see me suffer.
>
> Letty: That's not what she asked. You just want to play the victim all the time. Nothing is ever your fault and you do that so I will do all the work. Everything you do is a manipulation, just like you are doing now.
>
> Counselor: So, you both have some concerns about this process and are worried it won't work.
>
> Letty: He doesn't want it to work. He wants it to fail so I look like the bad guy in the relationship.
>
> Luis: I am the one who agreed to come. You just suggested it because you thought I would say "no" and then you could hang it over my head.

While Cluster I outline the characteristics of communication between high conflict partners, Cluster II: Hostile, Insecure Emotional Environment addresses the affective atmosphere created by these persistently negative and hostile interactions. In Anderson et al.'s (2011) model, Cluster II is defined by strong negative effects, emotional reactivity, lack of safety, mutual distrust, and triangulation. Once again, all couples experience the above issues to some degree at various points in the lifespan of the relationship, but for high conflict couples, these emotional reactions are firmly woven into the day to day experience of the relationship. While most relationships, when experiencing any of the above elements, might use that as a reason to change or seek help, high conflict couples see the negative emotional environment as normal, and if anything, blame the other partner (or outside forces) on the perceived struggle.

Counselor: In your description of your day to day life, it seems like most of your time is spent arguing and fighting.

Jackson: Don't all couples do that?

Counselor: In my experience, most couples are dissatisfied with the fighting and want to work to get the relationship to a place where it is more peaceful.

Jackson: They are probably lying to make you think they are nicer than they are. We are just real.

Kim: Yeah, we do fight a lot, but I think that's what couples do.

Jackson: It's mainly her attitude, so if we could do something about that, great.

Kim: Oh please ... you do your share of the fighting. In fact, I've never been in a relationship with anyone that seems to love to argue more than Jackson.

Jackson: I'm not arguing, I'm just stating my opinion. It's not my fault you are spoiled and can't listen to anybody but yourself.

An important characteristic of Cluster II is triangulation, and this concept will get more attention later in the book, but this is a good place to begin the exploration. High conflict couples are experts in pulling in outside professionals to take the blame from the couple.

Counselors are easy prey for triangulation because the traditional couples counseling set up creates a ready-made triangle (two clients, one counselor). Triangles are not designed to produce change but are arranged to remove stress temporarily from the couple. Unfortunately, if change is not the desired outcome, the triangle creates frustration and treatment failure. When caught in a triangle, counselors may feel they are struggling not to take sides and end up working harder than in a more balanced system. If the counselor sets boundaries, as they should, in high conflict couples, this often leads to the couple dropping out of counseling and searching for a more willing triangle participant. We will cover triangulation in-depth in later chapters in the book, as the avoidance of triangulation is a natural advantage of TCC.

Some Added Elements in of High Conflict Couples

The models of high conflict couples proposed by Gottman (1993) and Anderson et al. (2011) are useful in differentiating high conflict couples from other levels of relationship disruption. When we first began the formulation of TCC in early 2000, we utilized the available literature and our own experiences to help assess high conflict and work within the TCC approach to try and address these issues. In addition to the elements discussed, we came to identify a few other essential elements of high conflict. We will include them to round out the understanding of the high conflict couple experience.

Severe psychopathology in one or both members: Research shows that the rate for marital concordance, both partners having a diagnosable mental disorder, is very high (Galbaud du Fort, Bland, Newman, & Boothroyd, 1998; Hammen & Brennan, 2002; McLeod, 1995; Van Orden et al., 2012). The concordance of psychopathology is also connected to a higher level of marital discord, a decrease in marital functioning, and poor treatment outcome (Butterworth & Rodgers, 2008; Grant et al., 2007; Whisman, 2007; Whisman, Uebelacker, Tolejko, Chatav, & McKelvie, 2006). When couples enter counseling and severe psychopathology is present in one or both members, the level of relational dysfunction tends to be higher and more complex, calling for a need for quality assessment and a treatment that can be tailored to fit the needs of the clients.

Conflicting Family of Origin Patterns: Much like the other elements of high conflict couples, the differentiation among levels of conflict within couples is not distinguished by the presence of a conflicting family of origin patterns, but with the intensity and persistence of these issues within the relationship. For every relationship, each partner has a family of origin where the individual learned, through experience, the intricacies of relationships. This learning did not occur in isolation and therefore does not represent the totality of the person's relationship blueprint, but the nature of these early relationships—and the impact it has in the present—is worth investigating (Dreikurs, 1999). While most people are able to gain insight into their patterns and collaborate with their partner on a joining of the blueprints, high conflict couples either lack insight into their own patterns or hold rigidly onto their blueprint, unwilling to compromise. It is within the family of origin pattern search that many of the interaction breakdowns mentioned by Gottman (1993) occur. Consider these two summaries focused on the method for handling conflict in relationships and think about how the patterns would intersect:

Robert: I grew up in a large Italian family. My parents moved here from Sicily when they were 18. I have four brothers and two sisters, and we lived in a small brownstone in Brooklyn. When I think of conflict in my family, I would say it was in your face constantly. Everyone yelled all the time; if you didn't, no one would hear you. Every feeling was intense. I remember my mom saying we were "passionate" and that meant you cared. We didn't fight because we hated each other—we fought to show that we loved one another and sometimes it gets physical. I fought my brothers; I saw my dad put his hands on my mom several times. All that is unfortunate and I've worked hard not to do that in my relationships. But yelling? Oh yeah, anytime I get upset about something, I yell. How else are you supposed to let someone know you are upset?

Catherine: I grew up an only child in Nebraska. My mom was a stay-at-home mom and my dad worked in a bank. It was incredibly quiet at my house; I don't think I ever saw my parents fight. In fact, I would describe them as loving and happy, but I never really saw them talk about anything of substance. We ate dinner and the conversation was mostly on me; what I did that day and school. I remember one year, when I was 15, my maternal grandmother passed away. I don't think I saw either of my parents cry, not even at the funeral. My mom caught me crying in my room and told me to not waste any energy on that. It was always like we had to be in control of our emotions. I think people who get emotional are unsettled and abusive.

As you might be able to conclude, the opposite approaches to conflict and emotions could cause some disconnect within the relationship. Once again, it is important to note that it is not the presence of the pattern difference that is vital, but how the couple handles the difference. In a low conflict couple, the partners would learn about each other's approach and work together to forge a collaborative response to conflict and emotion, but high conflict couples rigidly believe that theirs is the best and only way and try to force it on their partner. Robert would characterize Catherine as uncaring and robotic, while Catherine would see Robert as abusive and out of control. They would resist meeting in the middle and see any attempt to compromise as a defeat; an indication that the way they grew up was unhealthy.

History of disturbed relationships: All people experience failure in relationships. In fact, if you look over your relationship history, every relationship (save your current), is technically a failure in that it was not sustainable, so it ended. Most people also recognize that an end to a relationship can also be a positive event. Even when a relationship termination is painful, the decision to move on can be a healthy choice. People who learn from their past relationships and adjust their general interpersonal strategies can also be viewed as using their relationship "failures" in positive and adaptive ways.

In high conflict relationships, it is typical for both partners to possess little insight into how past relationships impact their current functioning. In fact, when asked to talk about past relationships, we are often met with, "That's not really relevant" or "It's too painful to talk about. I was married to some really crazy people." The denial and blame approach to past patterns is a warning sign of possible high conflict. It is important to encourage exploration into this area as it will provide useful information about their approach to a wide array of relationship elements and allow the counselor with opportunities to build rapport. The difficulty will be in focusing the individual on their role in the relationship dynamic and not on the other person. The probe can be a vital platform in setting the counseling norm of focusing on self, instead of others, which will be an important dynamic as the counseling unfolds.

When high conflict couples open up about past relationship patterns, you will find consistency regarding the frequency and intensity of the high conflict elements. Getting a sense of the pervasiveness of the dysfunction is vital in the assessment of a high conflict couple and instrumental in introducing the importance of the patterns to the couple. I (K.A.F.) often use the metaphor of two rivers coming together as an example of a relationship formation. It starts with two rivers, each with its own flow path, and when the two rivers come together, it is seldom a calm, serene process. The joining produces turbulence, strange currents, and plenty of sediment, which clouds the water. Healthy couples are mindful of one's personal river and curious about the other's rhythm and flow of life. Each partner will use that history to gain a greater understanding of how the rivers come together to make one, with insight on how those patterns will create opportunities and threats within the relationship. High conflict couples have none of that insight or interest. They seem unaware of the dynamics of relationship formation, convinced that their approach to life is the right, if not only, approach. Patterns are important for understanding and improving relationships; they are even more important to understand in high conflict relationships. In healthy relationships, the patterns often work to enhance the relationship, but in high conflict couples, the intensity of the patterns will work to generate and preserve chaos in the relationship. To illustrate this difference between healthy conflict and high conflict couples, we provide an example, using the same pattern with different levels of insight and intensity.

Reggie and Melissa: Reggie's relationship history reveals a series of long-term (6 months to 2 years) relationships. Most of the time the relationships end because Reggie starts to lose interest in his partner: "It's like the passion drains out of the relationship." Once that happens,

Reggie begins to distance himself from the relationship and eventually breaks up. Melissa's history also contains mostly long-term relationships (1–4 years). Unlike Reggie, she never leaves a relationship. In fact, she reports that she has never broken up with a partner and is always the one getting "dumped." She notes that she can tell once a relationship is beginning to end but tends to "hang on at all costs" and does not do a good job at assessing whether the relationship is good for her.

Reggie and Melissa enter counseling with good insight into these patterns and are focused on what they want to do differently. Reggie states, "I think I have been passive about keeping the relationship alive. I have started noticing that dip in interest with my relationship with Melissa, and instead of expecting her to solve it, I think I want to take a more active approach in keeping the momentum. I want to be proactive and work with her to make the relationship better." Melissa observes, "I think with past relationships, I have been too reliant, almost desperate, for the relationship to work. I would be willing to keep quiet and keep the peace—anything to maintain the status quo. I want to do a better job of voicing what I want in the relationship. I have some great ideas and I want to take responsibility for stating my needs and working with my partner to being happy!"

Dirk and Desiree: Dirk's relationship history reveals a series of long-term (6 months to 2 years) relationships. Most of the time the relationships end because Dirk starts to lose interest in his partner: "It's like the passion drains out of the relationship." Once that happens, Dirk begins to distance himself from the relationship and eventually breaks up. Desiree's history also contains mostly long-term relationships (1–4 years). Unlike Dirk, she never leaves a relationship. In fact, she reports that she has never broken up with a partner but is the one to get "dumped." She notes that she can tell when a relationship is starting to end but tends to "hang on at all costs" and does not do a good job at assessing whether the relationship is good for her.

Dirk and Desiree enter counseling with little insight into these patterns and are focused on what the other person needs to do differently. Dirk states, "Desiree just doesn't do anything to add value to the relationship. She makes it so stale; I think I am just bad at finding the right partner. It's like, they get me on the hook and just stop trying. After a few months, she went into comfort mode and does nothing for me. I have been clear about what she needs to do to keep me around. If she isn't willing to meet my needs, I have no problem leaving and I've told her that several times; I am a good communicator. I have started noticing that dip in interest with my relationship with Desiree, and instead of expecting me to solve it, I think I want her to take a more active approach in keeping the momentum. She needs to be proactive and work to make the relationship better." Desiree observes, "I think with past relationships, I have worked really hard to make the relationship work. I don't really see a problem right now; I don't think he's unhappy. I don't really want anything to be different about our relationship. I feel like we work well together and are a solid team. I know he gets stressed out at work so I guess maybe I need to help him more with that, maybe not talk to him about my mom and just try to keep the peace a bit more. We just need to keep doing what we do and get through this life. Staying the course will create a sense of stability and that's what we need right now."

Severe social or vocational issues: Friendships can be a vital social support in relationships. Research shows that, in healthy couples, both men and women can benefit from discussing their relationship issues with friends and in most cases, the friend support adds to the commitment and positive growth direction in couples (Julien et al., 2000; Oliker, 1989; Proulx, Helms, & Payne, 2004). Sprecher (2011) noted that the social circle's positive view of the relationship also impacts the marital relationship in a positive manner. In a sense, the social network can act as a vital piece in the relationship feedback loop, adding positive and constructive opinions on the process, which can act as a key form of support for couples.

However, what happens when the feedback loop is pervasively negative, as in cases with high conflict couples? We have observed two consistent patterns: first, just as the social network acts to reinforce the positive flow in relationships, they will also tend to validate a persistently negative flow. When the negativity is one-sided and externalized, friends will validate and reinforce the predominant theme and support the friend's views. This acts to preserve the friendship but is not beneficial to the marital relationship. Second, there are many cases when friendship cannot bear the negativity and conflict and results in destruction; it is common for high conflict couples to report feeling socially isolated and being withdrawn from friends. They will rarely pinpoint the deterrence of their social networks to the conflict within the relationship and will often chalk it up as "we grew apart" or "they are too busy for me." Regardless, the high conflict robs the couple of the protective factor of supportive friends that is readily available to other couples.

Job-related stress can also have a negative impact on marital satisfaction and numerous studies have explored the relationship between vocational concerns and marital conflict (Crouter, Bumpus, Head, & McHale, 2001; Jackson et al., 2016; Perry-Jenkins, Repetti, & Crouter, 2000; and Story & Repetti, 2006). While these stressors can cause disruption in even the best relationship, they can magnify the chaos in a high conflict relationship. Work is often tied to financial security and can also be intensely perceived in high conflict couples. Much like the other elements, the distinguishing factor of a high conflict couple when it comes to job stress is their resistance to see the external threat (job loss, promotion, interpersonal work conflict, etc.) as a task to solve together and assess its impact and rehabilitation in solitary. They ignore the relational pathways and instead focus on defending and protecting themselves.

Unreasonable or rigid expectations of counseling: Lastly, in our experience, high conflict couples always come to us with two interesting counseling patterns. First, they always come with an extensive list of counseling failures. Like their previous romantic relationships, the patterns always focused on the counselor's lack of skill—with minimal liability given to the clients. In exploring the patterns in connection to how the couple approaches their treatment, you can often get a good sense of how these patterns are also reflected within the relationship.

Second, they always enter counseling with unreasonable or rigid expectations about counseling. This may manifest in beliefs that counseling will completely transform their relationship (if the counselor does it correctly), an oversimplification of the issues (i.e., communication), or an underestimation of the work that will be involved ("we only want to come once a month" or "can you give us a book and then we can call in and talk to you about it"). While setting realistic expectations is the beginning of every counseling journey, you will find that high conflict couples hold on to these beliefs stubbornly and persistently until the counseling creates sufficient boundaries and rapport to set new, productive boundaries. It is getting to that point in the process that makes high conflict couples so challenging. The following dialogue illustrates both types of unrealistic expectations:

Counselor: I see you have both been in individual counseling on and off over the years and even tried couples counseling a few times. What have you learned from these experiences?

Lila: It was a waste of money in my opinion. I really like individual counseling, but it's difficult for counselors to know all the ways to help.

Counselor: What do you mean?

Lila: Well, I'm into all sorts of things. I read a lot on the internet, so I consider myself somewhat of an expert on innovative treatments. I find it frustrating when I know more than the counselor about how best to help people.

Counselor: If they aren't up to speed and what you are researching, you lose faith in their ability to connect with you.

Lila: Oh, absolutely!

Rico: For me, it just seems to take so long. I mean, why do we have to come to counseling every week for, like, 30 years?

Counselor: Did you see someone in counseling for 30 years?

Rico: No way! I usually get frustrated after a couple of weeks and bail. I'm a busy guy and have lots of more important things to do. I must keep the money flowing for this one over here (points at Lila), so if it comes down to a counseling session or making money, I'm choosing money.

Counselor: I'm assuming that has gotten in the way of progress in the past counseling work.

Rico: Why do you call it work? I'm paying you to do the work. I'm here for the benefits and to get her off my back. But

> yeah, it seems to piss off counselors when I cancel sessions at the last minute. They don't seem to realize that my work comes first. This is like a side gig and quite frankly, I think you could move this along a little quicker. Sometimes I feel like counselors like to drag this stuff out just to make some extra money.

Domestic violence: Domestic violence is a serious societal issue that impacts millions of families every year. While there are occurrences of violence and abuse in all forms of couples—and some evidence of mutuality between partners—the research supports the conclusion that the vast majority of victims are women (Black, 2011; Breiding, Basile, Smith, Black, & Mahendra, 2015; Silverman, Decker, Reed, & Raj, 2006). Domestic violence is not a one-time behavior but represents a persistent and systematic cognitive and behavioral pattern of control within the relationship. This pattern will typically include high-intensity behaviors, such as physical and sexual abuse, but also include low-intensity behaviors, such as verbal abuse (name-calling, put-downs, silence, threats), emotional abuse (intense criticism, stalking, isolating other), and digital abuse (requiring access to passcodes, sending unwanted texts, controlling social media).

Domestic violence is rooted in the dynamics of power and control, and the manifestations and patterns that arise from these dynamics meet the criteria for high conflict. The field is split as to how best to treat the issue of domestic violence. While the couple's treatment has gained some support over the last few years (Simpson, Atkins, Gattis, & Christensen, 2008; Simpson Rowe, Doss, Hsueh, Libet & Mitchell, 2011; Stith, Rosen, McCollum, & Thomsen, 2004), many researchers and practitioners assert that treating domestic violence in traditional couples counseling puts the target of the abuse at an increased risk for violence (Bograd & Mederos, 1999; Christensen, Baucom, Vu, & Stanton, 2005; Gurman, 2008). In fact, Flasch et al. (2020), conducted an in-depth content analysis of the current state standards for Battering Intervention Programs and found that most states consider couples treatment a prohibited approach under state guidelines. Despite the field being concerned about treating domestic violence offenders outside of battering intervention groups, the likelihood of couples presenting in couples counseling with issues related to domestic violence is high, and the dynamics of domestic violence may make it difficult to discern at the beginning. We offer three crucial elements of domestic violence treatment that are important for your consideration as you assess your clients. When interacting with a couple experiencing domestic violence, please note:

1   It's all about power and control: The behaviors connected with domestic violence are designed for one primary purpose—to control their partner. This focus creates an obstacle of focusing on one's self, as the threat of lack of control is always seen as emanating from an external source. To mediate the internal feeling of threat, behaviors of power and control will be utilized within the relationship. More perceived threat equals more intense behaviors. This is often expressed as "If she would just do this, I wouldn't get so upset". While this external locus of control is common in most high conflict couples, not all choose the behavioral weapons of power and control.

2   Minimization, denial, and blame are high: To create some protection from the consequences of their actions, people who choose the method of power and control will mobilize a creative array of defenses. Minimization seeks to reduce the intensity or impact of the behavior by using "only" or "just" as modifiers. For example, "I only hit her once" or "I just pushed her out of my way" are common methods of reducing the gravity of the event, hopefully decreasing the consequence as well.

    Denial seeks to completely distance the person from the behavior, its impact, and the associated consequence. The defense can be profound. I (K.A.F.) have sat in front of an individual—with a police report and pictures of the damage caused by that individual—and have that person look at the documents and say, "They have it all wrong. I wasn't even at home that time". Denial also has the added consequence of making the other person feel like their version of reality is distorted, creating a pattern of self-doubt and second-guessing that can serve to reinforce the pattern.

    Blame is the most damaging of the defenses, as it places the responsibility on the victim. It is also problematic because it creates a system where wrong people are investing energy in solving the problem, which creates a cycle of failure, which leads to more blame (i.e., "You should try harder because whatever you are doing isn't working. I'm still upset"). As discussed in this chapter, blame is very destructive to the relationship and is common in high conflict couples.

3 The issue is commonly labeled "anger": A common presenting problem for couples experiencing domestic violence is anger. The perpetrator might say, "I have a minor problem with my temper" or the victim might say, "We have anger issues". Realizing the elements of minimization, denial, and blame will intrigue you about the anger and force you to explore deeper. Even in the way they describe the anger, utilizing some of the defenses mentioned earlier, provides some hints that there might be more to the story. For example, in the examples provided, when the counselor probes more into the anger, what she would commonly find is that the partner is assumed to be the cause, and is therefore expected to make the necessary adjustments for reconciliation. You might hear, "Yeah, she knows how to push my buttons" or "I have told her a million times, do not hassle me when I am in a bad mood. She knows what is going to happen if she does, but she does it anyway". In high conflict couples, efforts within the couple's counseling to localize the responsibility onto the person feeling the emotion will be met with fierce resistance. In relationships with domestic violence, it is important to recognize that this dynamic, although unhealthy, is employed to stabilize the relationship and maintain the pathway to relative peace, albeit maladjusted. The case example below highlights this dynamic:

Counselor: Fritz, tell me more about what your anger looks like.

Fritz: My anger? I don't know. I think it's pretty normal. I just get aggravated over normal things. Mainly Lucila, I guess ... she tends to piss me off more than most and she knows it. I think she does it sometimes just to get a rise out of me.

Lucila: I don't really like it when you get angry.

Fritz: Then why are you such a bitch all the time? I mean,

	seriously. You know what pisses me off and you do it anyway. Why can't you just leave me alone?
Counselor:	Fritz, let's refocus and be careful of the harsh name-calling. You seem to want to make Lucila responsible for your anger, but what if I threw out there the idea that you are responsible for the emotions you choose?
Fritz:	I would say that was a bunch of psychobabble! You mean to tell me that she can do whatever she wants, and I just take it and be happy? Maybe she can rub kitty litter on my face and I just sit there smiling and tell her she is great?
Counselor:	Well, not exactly. I...
Lucila (interrupts):	Yeah, I agree with Fritz. I get what he's saying. There are times when I just act all crazy. Maybe it's hormones, but I'll get on his case and I can get why he would get angry about that. That's not his fault.

In this example, not only does Fritz completely and aggressively avoid accountability for his emotions, but Lucila, sensing his increased intensity, rushes in to assume responsibility and calm him down. Within this framework, the couple's dynamics have a high probability of paralyzing traditional treatment formats.

4 Sharing produces more risk: In relationships with domestic violence, the dominant narrative will be focused on the victim taking the blame and responsibility for the issue, while the most intense violence will be held as a family secret. All counseling strives to create is an atmosphere of safety, where clients feel comfortable sharing aspects of themself and their relationship. If the victim buys into this illusion of complete safety and violates the norms of the relationship by sharing too much, the counselor cannot ensure that person's safety outside of the session. In fact, the counselor might not even know the impact of the revelation because the perpetrator will minimize the indignation, and the true extent of the behavior will not be evident until the couple returns home. The following

dialogue highlights how a counselor might unwittingly put their client in danger.

Counselor: Annie, I get the sense that there is more to the story about the argument you are discussing.

Annie: What do you mean? We had a disagreement about dinner. We talked about it and I started crying like a crazy person. I don't know why I do that. Anyway, we came to an agreement and moved on.

Counselor: Tell me more about the disagreement. What was your perspective and role?

Annie: I don't really remember. I was making steak and he said he didn't want steak. It was just a misunderstanding. We worked it out and I cooked fish instead. I don't know why I had to start crying and make a big deal out of it. I need to learn to not do that.

Counselor: How did Victor let you know he didn't want steak? And how did you voice your opinion about cooking steak rather than switching? I mean at that point; you were already cooking.

Annie: Well, he told me he didn't want steak. When I said I was almost finished cooking it, he .... um .... (fidgets) .... he called me an idiot and said he hated the way I cooked steak. He picked up one of the steaks and gave it to the dog.

Victor: Oh, come on. That's not what happened. She always makes a big deal out of nothing. She was cooking these cheap steaks and had burned the crap out of them. It was stinking up the whole house with the smoke. If we ate them, it would have been like eating leather. I told her we didn't have to eat them, no big deal, and offered to make the fish myself. She starts crying and ends up making the fish, even though I offered. The steak was inedible! I was trying to save her some trouble and this is the thanks I get.

Annie: You are right. I shouldn't have said anything about it.

> The message is subtle, but in this dialogue, Annie, at the counselor's urging shares more about the incident and violates the relationship norm. Victor steps in to smooth over the narrative, and all seems calm, but the counselor might not be aware of how this interaction might increase the possibility of violence after the session.

While the evidence of domestic violence might not be readily apparent, which makes the venture into couples counseling perilous, the unique advantage of TCC is that if the couple is assessed as high conflict and chooses TCC, they will each be moved into individual sessions where domestic violence dynamics can emerge more clearly. Once in individual sessions, the focus on the internal dynamics of each client can more effectively deal with the concerns mentioned above. Whether to continue to work with clients in TCC will depend on the frequency and intensity of the violence. It is appropriate to treat domestic violence issues in individual counseling if the issue of accountability is clearly defined and reinforced. If a referral is necessary, groups specifically designed to address battering intervention are available in most areas.

Summary

This chapter explored the various typologies and elements of a high conflict couple. Across all typologies and explanations, high conflict couples are differentiated from other couples by their persistent and intense behaviors, and attitudes that create discord in the relationship and make treatment much less effective. With this population in mind, TCC was formed. As you move through the remainder of the book, keep this population in mind and use the information in this chapter as a tool for assessing the couples you see in practice. Whether you use TCC or another approach, it is important to understand the unique challenges this population presents in the change process.

References

Anderson, S., Anderson, S., Palmer, K., Mutchler, M., & Baker, L. (2011). Defining high conflict. *American Journal of Family Therapy*, 39(1), 11–27.

Black, M. C. (2011). Intimate partner violence and adverse health consequences: Implications for clinicians. *American Journal of Lifestyle Medicine, 5*(3), 428–439.

Breiding, M. J., Basile, K. C., Smith, S. G., Black, M. C., & Mahendra, R. (2015). *Intimate partner violence surveillance: Uniform definitions and recommended data elements.* Retrieved from https://www.cdc.gov/violenceprevention/pdf/ipv/intimatepartnerviolence.pdf.

Butterworth, P., & Rodgers, B. (2008). Mental health problems and marital disruption: Is it the combination of husbands and wives' mental health problems that predicts later divorce? *Social Psychiatry and Psychiatric Epidemiology, 43*(9), 758–763.

Bograd, M., & Mederos, F. (1999). Battering and couples therapy: Universal screening and selection of treatment modality. *Journal of Marital and Family Therapy, 25*(2), 291–312.

Christensen, A., Baucom, D. H., Vu, C. T.-A., & Stanton, S. (2005). Methodologically sound, cost-effective research on the outcome of couple therapy. *Journal of Family Psychology, 19*(1), 6–17.

Cohen, O., & Levite, Z. (2012). High conflict divorced couples: Combining systemic and psychodynamic perspectives. *Journal of Family Therapy, 34*(4), 387–402.

Cohen, O., Luxenburg, A., Dattner, N., & Martz, D. (1999). Suitability of divorcing couples for mediation. *American Journal of Family Therapy, 27*(4), 329–344.

Crouter, A. C., Bumpus, M. F., Head, M. R., & McHale, S. M. (2001). Implications of overwork and overload for the quality of men's family relationships. *Journal of Marriage and the Family, 63*(2), 404–416.

Dreikurs, R. (1999). *The challenge of marriage.* Philadelphia: Accelerated Development.

Fall, K. A., & Howard, S. (2017). *Alternatives to domestic violence* (4th ed.). New York: Routledge.

Flasch, P., Haiyasoso, M., Fall, K., Evans, K., & Nesichi, T. (2020). A content analysis of the current state of batterer intervention program state standards. *Journal of Interpersonal Violence.* Manuscript submitted for publication.

Fraenkel, P. (2019). Love in action: an integrative approach to last chance couple therapy. *Family Process, 58*(3), 569–594.

Friedman, M. (2004). The so called high-conflict couple: A closer look. *American Journal of Family Therapy, 32,* 101–117.

Galbaud du Fort, G., Bland, R., Newman, S., & Boothroyd, L. (1998). Spouse similarity for lifetime psychiatric history in the general population. *Psychological Medicine: A Journal of Research in Psychiatry and the Allied Sciences, 28*(8), 789–803.

Gottman, J. M. (1993). The roles of conflict engagement, escalation, or avoidance in marital interaction. *Journal of Consulting and Clinical Psychology, 61*, 6–15.

Gottman, J. M., & Silver, N. (1999). *Seven principles for making marriage work.* New York: Three Rivers.

Grant, J. D., Heath, A. C., Bucholz, K. K., Madden, P. A., Agrawal, A., Statham, D. J., et al. (2007). Spousal concordance for alcohol dependence: Evidence for assortative mating or spousal interaction effects? *Alcoholism, Clinical and Experimental Research, 31*(6), 717–728.

Gurman, A. S. (Ed.). (2008). *Clinical handbook of couple therapy* (4th ed.). New York, NY: Guilford Press.

Hammen, C., & Brennan, P. A. (2002). Interpersonal dysfunction in depressed women: Impairments independent of depressive symptoms. *Journal of Affective Disorders, 72*(1), 145–156.

Jackson, G. L., Trail, T. E., Kennedy, D. P., Williamson, H. C., Bradbury, T. N., & Karney, B. R. (2016). The salience and severity of relationship problems among low-income couples. *Journal of Family Psychology, 30*(1), 2–11.

Julien, D., Tremblay, N., Belanger, I., Dube, M., Begin, J., & Bouthiller, D. (2000). Interaction structure of husbands' and wives' disclosure of marital conflict to their respective best friend. *Journal of Family Psychology, 14*(2), 286–303.

McLeod, J. D. (1995). Social and psychological bases of homogamy for common psychiatric disorders. *Journal of Marriage and the Family, 57*(2), 201–214.

Oliker, S. J. (1989). *Best friends and marriage.* Berkeley, CA: University of California Press.

Perry-Jenkins, M., Repetti, R. L., & Crouter, A. C. (2000). Work and family in the 1990s. *Journal of Marriage and the Family, 62*(4), 981–998.

Proulx, C. M., Helms, H. M., & Payne, C. C. (2004). Wives domain-specific "Marriage Work" with friends and spouses: Links to marital quality. *Family Relations, 53*(4), 393–404.

Silverman, J. G., Decker, M. R., Reed, E., & Raj, A. (2006). Intimate partner violence victimization prior to and during pregnancy among women residing in 26 U.S. states: Associations with maternal and neonatal health. *American Journal of Obstetrics and Gynecology, 195*(1), 140–148.

Simpson, L. E., Atkins, D. C., Gattis, K. S., & Christensen, A. (2008). Low-level relationship aggression and couple therapy outcomes. *Journal of Family Psychology, 22*(1), 102–111.

Simpson Rowe, L., Doss, B. D., Hsueh, A. C., Libet, J., & Mitchell, A. E. (2011). Coexisting difficulties and couple therapy outcomes: Psychopathology and intimate partner violence. *Journal of Family Psychology, 25*(3), 455–458.

Sprecher, S. (2011). The influence of social networks on romantic relationships: Through the lens of the social network. *Personal Relationships, 18*(4), 630–644.

Stith, S. M., Rosen, K. H., McCollum, E. E., & Thomsen, C. J. (2004). Treating intimate partner violence within intact couple relationships: Outcomes of multi-couple versus individual couple therapy. *Journal of Marital and Family Therapy, 30*(3), 305–318.

Story, L. B., & Repetti, R. (2006). Daily occupational stressors and marital behavior. *Journal of Family Psychology, 20*(4), 690–700.

Van Orden, K. A., Braithwaite, S., Anestis, M., Timmons, K. A., Fincham, F., Joiner, T. E., & Lewinsohn, P. M. (2012). An exploratory investigation of marital functioning and order of spousal onset in couples concordant for psychopathology. *Journal of Marital & Family Therapy, 38*(Supp S1), 308–319.

Whisman, M. A. (2007). Marital distress and DSM-IV psychiatric disorders in a population-based national survey. *Journal of Abnormal Psychology, 116*(3), 638–643.

Whisman, M. A., Uebelacker, L. A., Tolejko, N., Chatav, Y., & McKelvie, M. (2006). Marital discord and well-being in older adults: Is the association confounded by personality? *Psychology and Aging, 21*, 626–631.

3

PHILOSOPHICAL BASIS FOR A TANDEM COUPLES COUNSELING APPROACH

It might seem strange to have a chapter devoted to philosophy. In fact, you might be tempted to blow past these chapters altogether and get to the good stuff—the techniques, the case examples, and more of the hands-on aspects. We understand, but we also wanted to provide a place to explore the undercurrents that form the Tandem Couples Counseling (TCC) approach. During our time at Loyola New Orleans, a Jesuit university, we found that the environment inspired faculty who might not, under ordinary circumstances, explore the philosophical underpinnings of the subjects they teach. As evidence of this philosophical encouragement, Loyola University New Orleans included a three-hour graduate course entitled Philosophy of Counseling, even though most counseling programs do not have curricula that contain philosophy courses. By developing and teaching this course, we learned that counseling theories are vital, but philosophy provides a breadth of understanding that cannot be fully gleaned from counseling theory alone. The study of philosophy raises questions and offers possible answers to what it means to be a human being, the relative importance of relationships, and how we understand ourselves and others. Answers to these bigger questions can be particularly useful as we try to understand our clients' struggles and develop ways for them to improve their situations.

Now that we have hopefully interested you with the topic, we want you to know that this will not be the traditional discussion on philosophy you might expect in a text. We are not going to provide a survey of the most renowned philosophers and an overview of their works. In fact, we are not even going to explore general philosophy and tie the universal concepts to the treatment of high conflict couples. Instead, we are going to participate in the act of philosophy and explore some of the core concepts, dig a little deeper into what we think it means to be in a relationship, and what might be some critical elements of relating. Within this discussion, we will be looking at what we think about the nature of relationships and how the people within them make connections. Yes, we will also throw in some concrete philosophical terms to keep the discussion authentic.

Our habit of relying upon philosophy for one basis of understanding was repeated in the creation of this text. We explored the work of several philosophers and philosophy-oriented counseling theorists to help us identify and explore basic elements of relationships. While we could sit around and discover multiple philosophical roots and evolving branches that are embedded in the core of TCC, we decided to start the conversation with three central components: (1) intimacy, (2) meaning (how human beings understand or make sense of themselves and others), and (3) communication (how we convey our interpretations and misinterpretations to ourselves and to others). These concepts guided the development of TCC and formed its foundation, and each will be explored from a philosophical perspective. We hope this sort of journey will not only help illuminate some unexpected facets of your learning about TCC but also encourage you to do your own discovery process of your personal use of philosophy in your professional practice.

Intimacy

For couples, getting along, cooperation, respect, accountability, and responsibility are all essential elements, but they are not the destination.

We believe that the ultimate goal for successful couples is various forms of intimacy and all that these forms of engagement offered to couples. We will discuss intimacy in detail later in this chapter but at this point, it helps to explain that, depending on the couple intimacy, one or more of the following manifests: emotional, physical, and spiritual. By recognizing this priority and realizing the varied forms it takes, counselors are able to assist their clients better in developing goals and are made more conscious of the threats that may exist that could potentially derail their efforts. Unfortunately, modern society, with its ever-expanding array of technological advances, propels people toward isolation than interpersonal closeness. Isolation and loneliness now exist as chronic concerns that surface as easily in couples as they do in lone individuals. Human beings are social animals that require interpersonal contact to survive and achieve their potential. Learning to acquire and maintain such healthy relationships in an increasingly isolated setting can be challenging. Fortunately, the drive to seek out relationships resides within our biological dispositions.

Michael Kerr, a well-known psychiatrist and author, illustrates the intensity of the forces that cause human beings to seek out one another when he writes:

> The powerful ties that exist between family members are assumed to reflect instinctually rooted forces for emotional attachment that are part of mankind's mammalian ancestry. Cultures enact laws to discourage people from abandoning a spouse or children, but it is unnecessary to legislate attachment. Unless bad relationships have made a person wary of relationships, if he leaves or loses one set of attachments, he will seek new ones. Comfortably close connections activate brain chemicals that instill calmness and a strong sense of emotional well-being.
>
> (Kerr, 2008, p. 2)

Kerr's biological explanation for relationships and the benefit relationships offer provides a serviceable biological explanation of intimacy; his caution that those who are injured within relationships will be much less likely to pursue them is equally important. And it is important to realize that though history may make one less desirous of relationships, they are no less critical to a person's well-being.

Martin Buber, philosopher and author, offers an equally compelling perspective, though rooted in spiritual and philosophical assumptions about human beings rather than biological drives. Martin Buber's (1996) classic text "I and Thou" explores the vital role intimacy plays in the lives of human beings as it simultaneously explores spirituality and society. His obtuse writing style is challenging to read yet filled with profound insights and explanations. Many feel that the work is more poetry than prose, employing a style that speaks deeply to the reader's psyche. Remarkably, the process of reading the text often produces a powerful, palpable dialogue between author and reader. By way of example consider Buber's opening to Part 1:

> The world is two-fold for man in accordance with his two-fold attitude. The attitude of man is two-fold in accordance with the two basic words he can speak. The basic words are not single words but word pairs: one basic word is that word pair "I - You". The other basic word pair is the word pair "I - It"; ...
>
> Thus, the I of man is also twofold. For the "I" of the basic word "I - You" is different from that in the basic word "I - It."
>
> (Buber, 1996, p. 18)

In an ideal world, we would have preferred a lively and open discussion about the quote with the hope that the process would create a deeper level of understanding. Unfortunately, the following explanations of what may be gleaned from Buber's introduction will have to do. Buber maintains that human experience is either bound to objects (it) or to others (you). The author also stresses that the "I" relating to objects is different from the "I" relating to others. Human beings experience an inexhaustible sequence of "I - You" and "I - It" encounters throughout their lives. While Buber realizes that "I - It" encounters are common and necessary, the ability to experience both types of relationships enhances an individual's ability to understand the self as well as others. The human experience is such that continuous "I - You" cannot occur; such intense connections make repeated encounters impossible.

Simply interacting with another being does not define an "I - You" relationship. Individuals objectify people as they do inanimate objects or things. When clients complain that their spouses treat them more than the role they play in the family, they are experiencing the "It" in an "I - It" relationship—interacting with the I associated with the "I - It" rather than the I in the "I - You" with their spouse. The experience leaves them feeling used, discounted, isolated, and misunderstood. As you might suspect, objectifying others inhibits intimacy, while "I - You" relationships enhance it. Buber illustrates that important parts of self cannot be realized without "I - You" connections, but he also suggests that people cannot pursue such ways of relating; it occurs only when it is simultaneously allowed to happen. How they might know such a connection occurred comes to them only as a sense that something occurred, which allowed them to sense the depth and breadth of their spiritual, emotional, or physical connection. They recognize that boundaries between self and others briefly fell away and that they were connected to one another in a way that defies explanation.

This type of connection is rare, probably because it calls for two people to be in the same place at the same time. The location is often referred to as "The Ridge"—a place where boundaries that separate individuals briefly fall away and, in the process, create the necessary conditions for the "I - You." We believe that when Nin (2010) wrote, "Each contact with a human being is so rare, so precious, one should preserve it," she is referring to Buber's "I - You." In other words, we have many ways of relating to others but only one way of being intimately involved with them.

If such contact is so vital and important, why is it so elusive? According to Buber, progress and technological advances diminish the potential for "I - You." Modern life leans toward objectification than relation. One explanation is the fact that we are less interdependent on one another and therefore less likely to venture into the "I - You." Modernity reduces the need for occasions to relate. Aside from daily pressure of interdependence, predictable amounts of fear inhibit the effort to connect, especially fears born out of the need to be vulnerable and open to another in a way that allows "I - You" connections to occur.

What would people be afraid of? Why would they fear? How can they overcome the perceived threat? These are all reasonable and important questions to individuals wanting to overcome feelings of isolation and objectification, in a world where the drive to be close persists biologically, emotionally, spiritually, and physically. One plausible answer can be found in a discussion of the meaning and its importance to the health and well-being of individuals. The "I - You" encounter, because of the vulnerability generated, may spawn fears that may risk not only misunderstanding others but also themselves. The fear of losing one's self may be greater than the pain of isolation and loneliness. Such misunderstandings alarm people and generate fear of rejection as well as being hurt, taken advantage of, and seen as foolish. How we understand our interactions dictates, to a great extent, how willing we are to take the attendant risks to pursue them. With such a high premium placed upon the meaning, we rely on the work of Viktor Frankl to serve as an initial guide.

Meaning

Rooted in Existentialism, making meaning out of existence is seen as a primary part of life's journey and is manifested in the human tendency to structure and organize the countless stimuli experienced in any given day—over a lifetime—into a coherent, meaningful pattern or structure. This structure provides a context in which a person can pursue a chosen, and personally significant course of action; it eases anxiety and feels safe and comforting because it serves as criteria on how to live and feel significant.

The strive for meaning coexists alongside the element that produces the anxiety: meaninglessness. As Fall, Holden, and Marquis, (2017, p. 150) observed that meaninglessness stems from "the fact that objects of our perception do not have inherent meaning but only the meaning that, through an individual's own perceptual organization, one imposes on them—a meaning that, ultimately, the individual alone constructs. Rather, meaning in life, what one values, considers important or unimportant, considers being worthy or unworthy of one's pursuit and one's efforts is something humans create, both collectively and individually." As May and Yalom (2000) asked, "How does a being, oneself, another person, a client who requires meaning, find meaning in a universe that has no meaning?" (p. 286).

No better discussion of the importance of meaning to human experience can be found than in Viktor Frankl's (1963) now-classic work,

Man's Search for Meaning: An Introduction to Logotherapy. The very idea that people living in the most deplorable and restrictive conditions imaginable could persist in creating a meaningful existence, not only for themselves but for those they care about, exists as a compelling lesson to all. As a psychiatrist, Frankl was trained to assess and assist people in varied forms of psychological distress. What could have prepared him for what he was called upon to do within the confines of a World War II German concentration camp? Nevertheless, Frankl successfully created meaning and purpose for himself by working with others. By observing himself and many other prisoners he realized that those who created meaning in their lives sustained themselves, and those who did not perish. He documents the myriad ways people living in confinement discovered routes to meaning and purpose in settings that defied such efforts. The work serves as testimony to the strength that the search for meaning bestows upon people willing to make the journey.

According to Frankl, "Everyone has his own specific vocation or mission in life; everyone must carry out a concrete assignment that demands fulfillment. Therein he cannot be replaced, nor can his life be repeated; thus, everyone's task is unique as his specific opportunity to implement it." It is this uniqueness that forms both the call to create meaning and the recognition—how one creates meaning and purpose can never be the same as another's. In fact, according to Frankl, "Challenging the meaning of life is the truest expression of the state of being human." This task more than any other forms the essence of the human experience.

Frankl knows intimately well that, "Everything can be taken from a man or a woman but one thing: the last of human freedoms to choose one's attitude in any given set of circumstances, to choose one's own way." While we are not always able to choose the events that befall us, there is always the possibility that we can choose how to deal with them, and an attitude alone is not all we are left with. According to Frankl, "A human being is a deciding being," meaning, a person's life is fulfilled not only through attitudes, but also actions. Responsibility and accountability are philosophical cornerstones that form the goals of many counseling efforts. Frankl's sage advice guides the counseling process as well as directs individuals to create meaning and purpose within their lives: "When we are no longer able to change a situation - we are challenged to change ourselves."

The existentialists espoused that the primary pathway to change is through awareness and action. The specific elements of that awareness have some interesting philosophical roots applicable to our conceptualization of TCC. May (1961), in describing six aspects of being, outlined the conditions that help facilitate healthy awareness that allows for authentic meaning-making:

1 *Phenomenological centeredness* maintains that the best way to understand another person is through their own unique perspective—that human experience is best understood from the perspective of the individual. In order to get a clear sense of who my partner is, I must be willing to learn about what life means from her perspective, and the best way to learn that is to listen, be interested in that personal perspective, without foisting my beliefs and judgments onto them. In the same vein, I am the author of my life and determine what is and what is not meaningful to me. My responsibility is to own that part of my meaning-making and communicate my perspective to others to enhance their understanding of me.

2 *The potential to exist with other beings without losing centeredness* speaks to the importance of being able to form relationships with others and not lose one's sense of self. Buber's I-Thou relationship is a good example of this and will be explored more in the next section. In Figure 3.1 three types of relationships are illustrated. In the first set, the circles are set far apart from one another and the arrow denotes forces that push each entity away from the other. This would represent a relationship of extreme distance, where the meaning-making is so threatened by connection with another that the two choose distance as a mechanism for moderating this anxiety. In some situations, the elements of high conflict can produce a relationship dynamic of extreme disconnect where the meaning regarding relating is kept separate, out of fear.

The third set of circles represent the other extreme. In this relationship, only one definition of meaning is tolerated (the outside circle) and the arrows indicate the pressure to keep the other entity subsumed in the outer circle. In these relationships, the anxiety regarding meaning is so profound that the relationship operates under a belief system that is threatened by any difference in opinion of emotion. In an extreme

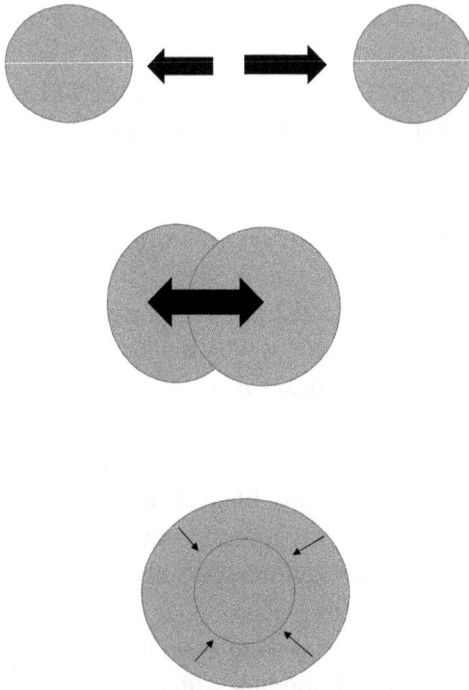

Figure 3.1 Three Relationship Models.

manifestation, the couple would think the same, feel the same, and act the same (like the same things, etc.). All things would be shared, and any individual form of meaning would be a threat and not tolerated. The dynamics of power and control, found in domestic violence, would operate within this relationship.

The second set of circles represent a healthy relationship dynamic and meaning-creation. In this relationship, the two circles are moderately overlapped, demonstrating shared connection as well as areas of individual identity. The arrows demonstrate the fluid back-and-forth motion of this relationship, honoring times when the relationship has more cooperation as well as times when the relationship moves apart, enjoying aspects of meaning that are separate from the relationship. In essence, a healthy relationship—one in which both partners honor the potential to exist without losing centeredness—will move along the continuum of circle connection illustrated in the figure, with the arrow denoting the movement being the only difference. The healthy relationship will move fluidly instead of rigidly moving apart or pushing one of the entities to be something they are not.

3 *Awareness as self-consciousness* allows the person to create meaning by sensing and integrating information about self through the utilization of internal and external processes. In a relationship, each partner can pursue meaningful aspects of life and assess those choices by how it makes them feel and receive feedback from others about their perception of those activities. Based on these two streams of feedback, the individual can make future choices on which creates the most meaning in life.

4 *Awareness as vigilance*, refers to the ability to sense and integrate information from one's surroundings to perceive threats to meaning and therefore, one's sense of self. It is important to realize that this perception is through a phenomenological frame, meaning that what is threatening to one might not be perceived that way by the other. The presence of vigilance is not the problem; in fact, it is an essential element for healthy functioning. The key is what the individual and the relationship do with their respective vigilance. If one member perceives a threat to meaning, do they disconnect or seek to understand its nature, and use the relationship to process what is uncovered? High conflict couples unilaterally employ destructive forces to deal with the threat. As discussed in Chapter 2, the elements of high conflict erode and obstruct the relationship's ability to address concerns and evolve.

5 *Anxiety as the struggle against non-being:* From an existential perspective, anxiety is the normal response to living. When one considers the process of meaning-making in life, the anxiety is felt when one ponders the lack of meaning in day-to-day choices. Haven't you ever thought to yourself, "Today was a total waste of time" or "I don't like my job. I just feel like I'm not living up to my potential"? When you have these thoughts, anxiety begins to creep in and, in most cases, fuels thoughts of how meaningful your day or job was, or motivates you to do something different (i.e., make a plan to be productive and look for a new job).

In relationship, anxiety related to the process and development of the relationship are also normal. "Is he the one?", "Is having a baby the next step for us?", or "Am I happy in this relationship?" all generate some anxiety because the answers define the relationship and greatly impact the next set of choices. All of this is normal—when anxiety is used to motivate, rather than paralyze. Consider the following two examples of the use of anxiety within a relationship:

Greg comes home one evening and says to Eliza, "Hey, I've been feeling like we have been in a rut lately. We seem to sit around every weekend and just watch television. How about we sign up for some ballroom dance lessons? It might be fun." Eliza considers the request and feels anxious over his statement about being in a rut. She begins to feel like Greg is saying he is dissatisfied with being in the relationship and therefore is dissatisfied with her. As her anxiety begins to build, her thoughts race and she concludes that Greg doesn't even want her to go to the ballroom dance lessons; he knows she won't want to go. He is hoping she says no so he can go by himself or take that new girl from work he has been talking about lately.

Greg comes home one evening and says to Eliza, "Hey, I've been feeling like we have been in a rut lately. We seem to sit around every weekend and just watch television. How about we sign up for some ballroom dance lessons? It might be fun." Eliza considers the request and feels anxious over his statement about being in a rut. She notices the anxiety and takes a moment to assess what else it could be about. She has been feeling a little stagnant in the relationship, but that's not necessarily a terrible thing; it is comfortable and there is some safety in it. However, Greg is feeling it as well, so maybe she can do something about it. She wants excitement in the relationship and although she is a little scared and anxious to try something new, she decides to try it.

In the first example, Eliza's anxiety moves her in a negative direction, which will also move her away from Greg. She feels threatened by his observation of the relationship and perceives the anxiety as a confirmation that something is desperately wrong with her and the relationship. In the second example, she takes the anxiety and considers several ways of dealing with it. Instead of using it in an adverse manner, she manages it, propelling her to try something new that will also potentially be beneficial to the relationship.

6 *Courage to self-affirm* is the process and ability to embrace the ways that one creates meaning in life, to enjoy the choices made, and be excited about the power that comes from being able to define one's existence. In relationships, this works the same way. Both partners respect the autonomy of the other and are genuinely interested in how their partner consciously makes sense of the world. This curiosity encourages the couple to explore overlaps in the meaning-making process, and the ways that their partners establish an identity outside of the relationship.

Couples' counseling, especially from a TCC perspective, undertakes the challenge of exploring meaning by recognizing that changing a relationship can change the couples themselves. Couples must create meaning—not only of themselves but also within the context of their relationship—to be successful. They are responsible not only for themselves but also for the relationship they create. Of course, creating meaning is no simple task. Such struggles are renowned and so common that they often become the humor in conflict within couples. References to the "battle of the sexes," inherent difficulties in getting one gender to understand and communicate effectively to the other exist in many formal and informal settings.

This discussion of meaning and purpose offers a glimpse into why people find intimacy threatening. The fears associated with intimacy may develop because such close encounters can easily threaten meaning as well as purpose. Overwhelmed and feeling lost without solid definitions of who we are and how we are, we seek the protection that defensiveness and rigidity offer. Unfortunately, such experiences and reactions lead towards misunderstanding, confusion, and conflict, and away from the intimacy so critical to the couple's relationship. To be successful, such encounters require a deeply developed sense of self; however, this comes about through intimate encounters. In order to be helpful to clients, counselors need to have some idea about the way human beings create meaning (as well as a misunderstanding), recognize how difficult it is to arrive at shared meanings, and develop a route to helping individuals relate to others in ways that tend to increase meaning, purpose, and ultimately, intimacy. To aid in developing this aspect, we turn to the Philosophy of Interpretation. Relying on this philosophical approach allows us to understand interpersonal communication and the role more fully as it plays in the creation of meaning and intimacy.

Communication

Hermeneutics, a philosophy of interpretation, suggests that individuals create meaning through an identifiable but complicated process. Hermeneutics also offers a promise that inspires us to endure as we pursue the arduous journey of understanding so that we come to grasp the meaning in our own lives as well as in others. We open with this quote from (http://plato.stanford.edu/entries/hermeneutics/ Hermeneutics First published Wed Nov 9, 2005) Obtained 3/12/10 describing how difficult it is to understand another.

> Here, Derrida questioned the idea of a continuously unfolding continuity of understanding. Meaning, he insisted, is not based on the will to dialogue alone. Most fundamentally, it is made possible by absence, by the relations of a word to other words within the ever-evasive network of structures that language ultimately is. Our relation to the speech of others, or to the texts of the past, is not one of mutual respect and interaction. It is a relationship in which we have to fight against misunderstanding and dissemination, one in which the focus on communality in language provides but a harmful illusion.

Here, hermeneutics suggests the possibility of a very complete level of understanding accomplishable not only in the dialogue between people but also through written communication. This understanding of the other—whether an individual with whom we are engaged in dialog or an author whom we read—offers us the potential to expand what we understand of ourselves as we discover and explore meaning in others. The philosophy wisely cautions that misunderstanding haunts both forms of interaction, dialogue and reading. Language can fool us into believing that we mean the same things when we use the same words. However, words are not meaning; to be accurate, meaning must be developed through dialogue—a complicated process where reciprocity, the give and take in dialog, becomes fundamental to the process of seeking meaning.

Such communication difficulties are equally well-known to people less versed in philosophy. For example, when couples summarize their difficulties as a "communication problem" (and many do), they are letting you know how unsuccessful they have been in the fight against "misunderstanding and dissemination;" when couples endure trust-eroding experiences that may cause them to say "I cannot believe you" or "Those are just words and not how you really feel," they are struggling with confusion borne out of the difference between what one says and how one acts. Once trust falls away, couples experience predictably intense emotions—those that rapidly cloud meaning and strain the ability to communicate effectively. Pain and fear dull efforts to understand and participate in meaningful dialogue. Unable to success-fully contain these emotions, couples often seek outside support. Relatives, friends, counseling professionals, or all three may be brought into the conflicted relationship.

Unfortunately, at this point, couples pursue outside support for rea-sons that tend to obstruct rather than enhance intimacy; each of the couples searches for an ally. Rigidity and defensiveness limit the ability to develop deeper understandings. They would rather be right than open themselves to the possibilities that new meaning and intimacy offer. Distress creates a desire for "The Truth." If they are right and the other is wrong, the tension somehow decreases even though no universally defined truth exists for the issues most couples struggle with.

The Truth

The pursuit of truth has always been a bit of a sticky prospect, but it is particularly difficult in counseling and even more troublesome in couples counseling. The dilemma is magnified exponentially when dealing with a high conflict couple. As Sullivan (2008, p. 193) explains:

> I am interested in a much more pragmatic and experiential sense of truth. These are truths that are founded on personal belief and an emotional connection (e.g., God's existence). It is my contention that these kinds of deep beliefs or truths invest dialogue with meaning,

value, and emotion. Reciprocally, however, they are also truths that emerge from the particular kind of dialogue we are having. For instance, in a heated argument with the other, the truth of what we are saying may become even more entrenched and indisputable.

Ironically, the moment that dialogue becomes most important for the couple, it becomes most difficult to accomplish. The couple invests energy in convincing the other at exactly the time they should be applying as many resources as they must understand.

Sullivan (2008, p. 194) writes:

There is a dynamism to the embodied, experiential space we construct through language as we vie to have our own particularly truth emerge victorious.

We may become increasingly strangled, may end up confessing that we are on the verge of tears, or begin to inwardly mock our friend's comments. In all these cases, there is an interesting relationship between the form of our dialogues, the kinds of truths we are attached to and our sense of self.

Certain topics, though vital to the relationship, produce reactions that blunt efforts to relate, obstruct dialogue, and interrupt the ongoing pursuit of creating meaning within the relationship. In general, the vagaries of language and idiosyncratic meaning contaminate the process of understanding—shift to an emotionally charged topic, and the need and ability to understand begin to vary inversely. What couples need most is exactly what they are least able to create. A model outlining the process and identifying how individuals can overcome the resistance offers some hope to struggling couples and those who wish to help them.

Spiral of Interpretation

One way of operationalizing concepts found in hermeneutics, so that couples can be helped more readily, can be found in "The Spiral of Interpretation," Michael Cowan's (1995) graphical description of how meaning and behavior are related to one another. As you can see, the model charts the relationship between various cognitive and behavioral aspects of human experience. His work focuses on how assumptions, interpretations, actions, and the reactions of others collectively influence an individual's thoughts and behavior. The model also identifies how and where change is possible as well as why change is so difficult.

Cowan (1993) stresses that "real" conversation dramatically affects our understanding of the world and the assumptions that we hold about ourselves and others. He references some simple but useful rules:

> Conversation is a game with some hard rules: say only what you mean; say it as accurately as you can; listen to and respect what the other says, however different or other; be willing to correct or defend your opinions if challenged by the conversation partner; be willing to argue if necessary, to confront if demanded; to endure necessary conflict; to change your mind if the evidence suggests it.
>
> (Tracy, 1987, p. 19)

And, most importantly, he suggests that we summon the courage to listen as completely as we can to others. He urges us not to fear that our silence while listening will be misconceived for agreement. At the same time, he understands how difficult it is to suspend judgment—the necessary precursor to the act of listening—when discussing issues where we have a great deal at stake. His work describes why relationships can be so challenging and, at the same time, critical to health and well-being.

Simple but Powerful

The Spiral of Interpretation (see Figure 3.2) begins by identifying "Background Understandings or Basic Assumptions." In everyday language, we might ask someone "What's your take on things?" or, "What's it like in 'your world'?" Anthropologists might use the term "World View" while psychologists might call such basic assumptions "Schema." Regardless of the term used to refer to assumptions, it is important to realize their profound influence. Clients experience no difficulty understanding the concept and using it. When they refer to their spouse's family and say something like, "You know, the Joneses' are like that" they are referring to a set of assumptions common, in this case to their in-law's family pattern.

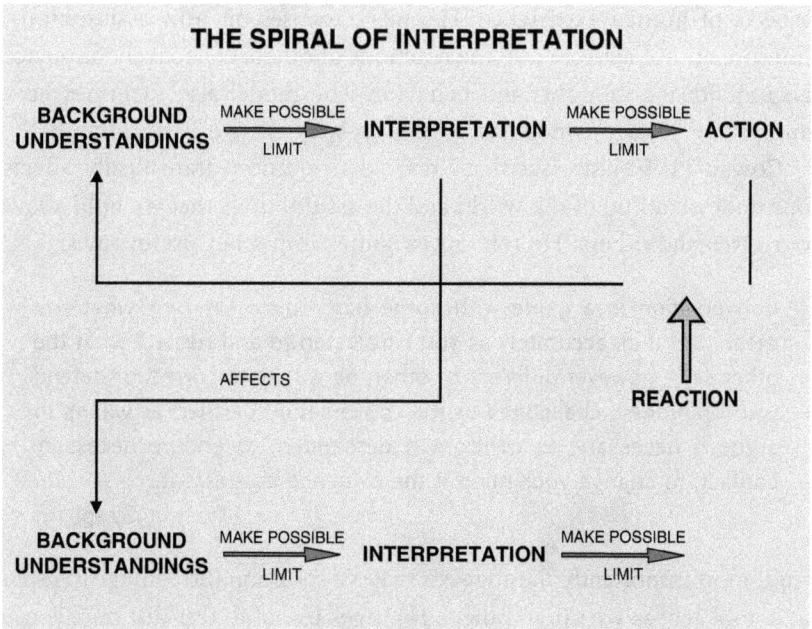

Figure 3.2 Spiral of Interpretation Cowan (1995).

These basic understandings affect the way we interpret events and how we act, how others react to us, and the meaning we create from our experiences. To be specific, basic assumptions make some interpretations possible and others impossible. For example, if one of our basic assumptions is that others are irresponsible, we will interpret offers of help from another very differently than if we believe people tend to act responsibly. Such interpretations influence the actions we take, allowing some and hindering others. We are not likely to take someone up on an offer of help if we interpret the offer as empty and unlikely to be carried out. Eventually, whatever actions we take will be reacted to by others. And their reaction will influence our background understandings.

If for example, a wife makes a good faith offer to help her husband and, having a set of background understanding from years with his dysfunctional family, he responds to his wife's offer with suspicion, distrust, and sarcasm, her help is likely to be withdrawn and he unwittingly hampers what she was trying to repair. These unfortunate background understandings are reinforced, and the couple's distress expands. On the other hand, if the offer is accepted gracefully, and the husband is helped by the wife's efforts, the background understandings will change, and their level of intimacy will increase.

As you can see, this process, for better or worse, links background understandings to interpretations, actions, and eventually to the reactions of others. It also contains the potential for change at each of the stages. Specifically, individuals may remain fixed or they may begin to explore new background understandings, thereby changing their interpretations and eventually allowing the creation of new behaviors. The spiral is a continuous process, and each step offers both the possibility for change and an opportunity to validate the problems within the relationship.

This model encourages us to perceive a couple as two individuals from two distinct cultures. Each has its own set of background understandings and a host of patterns—some that coincide with their mate and others that exist in stark contrast. Imago Therapy offers a useful perspective on these differences by implying that couples select one another because they are different people and that these differences are potentially complementary. In other words, each member of the couple is expected to resolve their idiosyncratic conflicts through a relationship with someone who has mastered what troubles the other.

This reciprocity and its promise of greater internal peace attract people to each other yet learning to use such opportunity can be quite difficult. The status quo, though unpleasant, is often preferable than the risk of changing the basic understandings that we have developed over a lifetime, and upon which we rely for the meaning that is important in making sense of our lives and relationships. Fear of change and of the unknown often combine to make the couple's journey difficult and perilous.

We have found that couples in conflict often fall to predictable patterns in their relationship history. For example, one couple reported that when problems develop, they would respond by going in what they called "opposite directions." The husband always went to his study and used the computer. We called it "isolating" and they instantly agreed with the term. The wife followed him wherever he went and kept insisting that they talk about what was happening; we called this "pursuing" and they also easily approved of this term. Armed with language that labeled their behavior (isolating and pursuing), we asked them to help us understand the background that caused them to select this pattern as a reaction to stress. They easily explained why they were doing it but had trouble understanding why it was disturbing for their respective partners. The husband said he needed time alone to think and felt that talking would only make it worse; the wife said she pursued because couples need to "talk things out" and added that if they stopped talking, it would signal the demise of the relationship.

You can easily estimate the source of these background understandings by imagining what their respective family of origin lives were like. Depending on how you look at it, they were both correct—couples both need time to talk and be alone. Based on the philosophical perspective we are considering, the most important thing that they were missing was the effect these patterns were having on their ability to establish and benefit from the chain of "I—You" encounters that were seriously missing in their life as a couple.

They needed a way to manage the fears that their assumptions and interpretations were creating for them. The exploration of their individual assumptive worlds proved to be an important first step. The husband eventually recalled seeing his father "pestered" repeatedly by his mother. The wife easily remembered her mother straining under what she called her father's "silent treatment." According to Anais Nin, "We don't see things as they are, we see them as we are." Armed with alternative interpretations of the very behaviors that once produced extreme levels of anxiety, the couple began to allow significant changes in their background understandings of what one another's behavior meant to each and to their relationship. Eventually, the couple worked out a productive response to stress where each member's needs, as well as those of the relationship, was met. The husband no longer saw his wife as pestering and the wife no longer saw her husband as retreating from the marriage. Once the fears of being pestered or abandoned softened, the couple honored their relationship needs for time alone and time together.

At this point, all the couple needed to cement the change to their individual assumptive worlds was an affirming reaction from the outside world—one that confirmed the benefit of seeing one another differently and acting with a greater tolerance for one another's concerns. Remarkably, that confirmation came from their children. Seeing parents cooperate, respect, and do the best they could to understand one another calmed the children and freed them to participate more fully and productively at home and in school.

With the affirmation of their children reinforcing the changes to each member of the couples' assumptive worlds, they discovered that a much deeper and more empathetic understanding existed between them. They sensed one another's pain and happiness in a way that caused a bond that previously did not exist. By changing their basic assumptions, they embarked on a set of behaviors that eventually allowed them to replace the "I - It" saturated relationship with which they were struggling with enough "I - You" encounters to spawn the intimacy that both unknowingly missed and now cherished. The effect on the family was so palpable that the couple was left with little choice but to pursue a course of closeness—not only with themselves but also with other members of their family. Over time, they came to understand that they had other choices than those that recreated the same suspiciousness and dysfunction that inhabited their respective families of origin,

Summary

In this chapter, we asked that you consider the possibility that the overarching goal of couples' counseling should be intimacy, though abstract—focusing much more on what exists between the couple and less on what exists within each member of the couple. We also suggested that pursuing this goal, clinicians would need to be concerned with how clients create meaning in their lives and how they communicate what they know and feel with each other. Martin Buber's work illustrated that a couple's intimacy occurs on one or more of three basic planes: emotional, spiritual, and physical. We also stressed the fact that human beings regularly, and quite appropriately, objectify one another to accomplish tasks, control their fears, and meet the challenges of daily life. We demonstrated that technological advances, coupled with the stresses of modern daily life, severely limit intimacy opportunities. In Buber's terms, opportunities for "I - You" encounters became so rare that couples were unable to establish sufficient levels of intimacy. Without such encounters, couples tend to fall into a maladaptive cycle with the very same problems they grew up in. The opportunity to allow their marriage to heal them from the wounds that they encountered through their lives is lost in a particularly painful way. The opportunity to be healing to one another is replaced with actions that are additionally injurious to the couple and to their relationship.

We also outlined how challenging it can be for a couple to explore the basic assumptions that guide their life choices and the way in which they make sense of events. Confusion about assumptions and difficulties in communicating ideas, feelings, and expectations combine to make life difficult for the couple and challenging for therapists who want to be helpful to them.

The philosophically broadened view of couples counseling offers unique insights into better ways to understand conflict and improved strategies for helping couples become healthier and more peaceful. Perhaps the most important conclusion that we drew from this philosophical journey was the overarching need to focus, at times almost myopically, on the relationship between the couple and not the people who form the relationship. Aligning with their relationship also proved to have many important positive effects during TCC. Remarkably, this unique focus allowed us to understand that one of the healing effects could be found in the way the relationship between the two counselors positively impacted the relationship between the couple. More about this interesting perspective and examples will be provided in the remaining chapters.

References

Buber, M. (1996). *I and thou.* New York: Touchstone.

Cowan, M. A. (1993). The sacred game of conversation. *The Furrow*, 44, 30–34.

Cowan, M. A. (1995). *Sociocultural context of ministry.* New Orleans, LA: Institute for Ministry, Loyola University.

Fall, K. A., Holden, J. M., & Marquis, A. C. (2017). *Theoretical models of counseling and Psychotherapy* (3rd ed.). New York: Routledge.

Frankl, V. E. (1963). *Man's search for meaning: An introduction to logotherapy.* New York: Pocketbooks.

Kerr, M. E. (2008). Why do siblings often turn out very differently. In A. Fogel, B. J. King & S. Shanker (eds.), *Human development in the twenty-first century: Visionary ideas from systems scientists.* Boston: Cambridge University Press.

May, R. (1961). *Existential psychology*. New York: Random House.

May, R., & Yalom, I. D. (2000). Existential psychotherapy. In R. J. Corsini & D. Wedding (Eds.), *Current psychotherapies* (6th ed., pp. 273–302). Itasca, IL: F. E. Peacock.

Nin, A. (http://www.brainyquote.com/quotes/quotes/a/anaisnin162996. html) Obtained 4/17/10.

Sullivan, P. (2008). Our emotional connection to truth: Moving beyond a functional view of language in discourse analysis. *Journal for the Theory of Social Behaviour, 38*(2), 193–207.

Tracy, D. (1987). *Plurality and ambiguity*. San Francisco, CA: Harper & Row.

4

CO-THERAPY
Rationale and Effective Application

Blake was excited to begin the clinical portion of his graduate training. While the content courses on theory, ethics, and other topics were interesting, he longed to put that information into practice with actual clients. He was most anticipating working with couples. As he looked at the intake roster, he was pleased to see that he was assigned a couple as his first client. He also noticed something peculiar: another counselor's name appeared next to his. What could this mean? He asked his supervisor and she remarked that he would be doing co-therapy with Kim. Co-therapy? What was that? He had never heard of that before outside of group class. To make matters more complicated, he did not know Kim. Blake's enthusiasm turned into anxiety as he realized he would be doing something he did not feel comfortable with someone he didn't know.

Blake's experience is common for beginning mental health professionals. It is not surprising for co-therapy to be used in the training of counselors, and although it is frequently used in group counseling, it can also be found in marriage and family training programs (Hendrix, Fournier, & Briggs, 2001). As individuals are trained in a modality such as co-therapy, they take the experiences and translate them into their evolving sense of meaning working with that approach, and foundational experiences become the frame for future practice. Therefore, having a good sense of the nature and purpose of co-therapy becomes crucial to the practice and its impact on the therapeutic process. The next section seeks to define co-therapy and provide a comprehensive definition that will help guide the use of the modality within Tandem Couples Counseling (TCC).

What is Co-therapy?

A simple consideration of what constitutes co-therapy might lead one to conclude it is merely a therapeutic environment where more than one mental health professional works on a client or group of clients. In this definition, the critical element is the number of counselors, but we believe co-therapy has always been intended for more. Roller and Nelson (1991) define co-therapy as "A form of psychotherapy in which the relationship between co-therapists becomes a crucial factor in the change process" (p. 3). This definition identifies the *relationship* as the focus and clinical rationale for choosing the specific modality of co-therapy. As you will learn throughout the remainder of the text, the co-therapy relationship can be explored and utilized in sessions with clients, consultations with one another, and supervision. While the general dynamics of co-therapy is covered in this chapter, it is always with the focus on the importance of the relationship and how to maximize its potential in the service of the clients. The use of the relationship, unique to TCC, is further explored in the following chapters of the book.

When one works diligently to develop the co-therapy relationship, the team will be utilizing the modality as intended, and the benefits of the approach will be most attainable. In their research of co-therapy practices, Roller and Nelson (1991, p. 15) articulated five main benefits of co-therapy, when the relationship is an identified instrument of change:

1   A greater opportunity for learning through discussion and collaboration: Co-therapists who are committed to the developing relationship learn and improve skills by watching the other therapist work and have an opportunity to learn about their own therapeutic

selves by being open to feedback. This interchange enhances the skill set of each counselor while also improving the co-therapist bond through the increase in vulnerability, trust, and respect.

2   Widened perspectives for therapists: While it is also mentioned in this chapter that co-therapy teams work best when working from compatible theoretical positions, this means that the theories need to be philosophically congruent, not that the theories must be identical. Working with someone from a different theory can help stretch your knowledge of the theory and can deepen understanding of how other perspectives explain client dynamics. In fact, it is within these theory divergences that the co-therapy team can begin to experiment with being comfortable with differences, and communicating and negotiating the mediation of the natural variance in beliefs about self, other, the work, and the clients.

3   Widened transference possibilities for clients: Although transference is a psychodynamic theoretical concept, co-therapists from every theoretical foundation can understand that clients will be responding and interacting with the counselors based on deeply-ingrained inter and intrapersonal patterns of relating. With two counselors, the clients have more people to interact with—both at the individual and relational level (client-counselor and counselor-counselor pairs). These experiences and reactions can be used to gain awareness into patterns of relating and can be the foundation for change.

4   Greater learning opportunities for clients: As the benefits for therapists are realized, the impact can also be felt by the clients. With two counselors, the clients are not limited by the skill threshold of a single counselor. Instead, weaknesses in one counselor can be overcome by relative strength in the other.

5   Opportunity for a checks and balances system for therapist behavior: When there is only one therapist in the room, there is little oversight of the process. No matter how much the therapist wants to be egalitarian in the approach with the clients, the therapist still largely controls the flow and focus of the work. With two counselors who are working together inside and outside the session, the opportunity to catch aspects of the work that are

outside one person's awareness is increased. A fully functioning co-therapist relationship also relies on feedback, which enhances the focus and flow of the counseling.

In reviewing marriage and family literature, it is not always apparent that co-therapy was studied with an eye on the relationship as the therapeutic mechanism. In fact, most of the research and commentary focused on the hypothesized benefits and consequences of the use of multiple therapists, and whether co-therapy is best utilized as a training tool or should be reserved for similarly skilled professionals (Fall & Menendez, 2002; Hendrix et al., 2001; Roller & Nelson, 1991). Unfortunately, most of the research on co-therapy does not take into consideration the impact of the co-therapy relationship. For example, Mehlman, Baucom, and Anderson (1983) specifically studied the impact of co-therapy when compared to individual treatment with couples, but the methodology only focused on client outcome and provided no emphasis on the relationship between co-therapists. Ellickson and Seals (1986) studied gender roles in co-therapy with a premarital couple, but never mentioned the role of the co-therapy relationship on the counseling process. In fact, the stated reason for choosing co-therapy had nothing to do with the relationship—an attempt to use two gender theories with the client.

In addition to the lack of attention, the relationship seems to get when researching co-therapy, also absent in discussions is how to best utilize co-therapy. In marriage and family literature, the two principal areas of exploration are training applications and co-therapy teams with congruent levels of skill. Co-therapy is often proposed as a useful method of training counselors as it either provides support (for both neophyte pairs) or in vivo supervision (one seasoned clinician and the other a student). Interestingly, Roller and Nelson (1991) do not consider either pairing as an example of co-therapy because in the neophyte pairing, neither is an experienced therapist and in the supervision example, the relationship is not between peers, so the inequality distorts and defines the relationship. This criticism of the use of co-therapy for training is common in the field. Jay Haley, one of the more well-known marriage and family therapists remarked, "I believe that using co-therapy in training only teaches the trainee to sit back and watch the teacher work" (1996, p. 19).

While the criticism of using co-therapy as a training method is well documented, there are those who have explored and detailed the possible benefits (Hendrix et al., 2001). The key is how the team, regardless of the set-up, utilizes the relationship. Consider the two training examples below:

Julie is excited to begin her internship and work with couples. She is told that for her first month, she will be paired with her supervisor in a co-therapy model while working with three couples. Her supervisor meets with her prior to the first sessions and informs her that she is to observe his work with the couples for the first month. She is to not say anything during the sessions but will have time to process the cases with him after each session. During the sessions, Julie sits quietly and observes her supervisor. At one point in the third session, Julie reflects a feeling expressed by one of the clients and her supervisor reminds her to "please refrain from interrupting and focus on observation for now."

James is eager to begin his advanced clinical work with couples. The site offers co-therapy as an option and encourages James to interview the senior staff to see if there is anyone who would be a good fit for him. After meeting with several people, James and Hannah, a staff psychologist, agree to work together in two cases. Hannah offers to meet with James before the first session and they discuss their initial views of the clients and openly process their feelings (anxiety, hope, etc.) about working together. Hannah mentions that there is an inherent power differential between them, and they explore how that might impact the work. They decide to make sure to check in with one another during the session and be available to process afterward. During the first session, Hannah notices James is being quiet and checks in with him by saying, "James, I notice you have been listening intently the past five minutes. I'm interested in what you are thinking."

1   What are the major differences between the two training scenarios? What is the role of the supervisee? The role of the supervisor?
2   How do the separate roles impact the training?
3   How do you think the distinct roles would impact the work with the clients?

As one examines the existing literature on co-therapy, a glaring omission seems to emerge; the core of the rationale for using co-therapy—the therapeutic impact of the relationship—has been left out of this exploration. It reminds us of trying to use a bicycle without using the pedals. Can a bicycle work without the pedals? Yes. We can push the bicycle; we can carry the bicycle. But do either of these utilize the true potential of the bicycle? No. In the same way, clinicians can certainly use co-therapy without considering the relationship, but these clinicians will be missing out on the real potency and purpose of co-therapy in the first place—to use the relationship as a means for change. As McMahon and Links (1984, p. 385) stated, "Therapists who are of the opinion that the co-therapy relationship has minimal therapeutic value fail to understand the potential for this type of therapy."

Once we realize that the quality of the relationship can greatly impact the potency of the co-therapy modality and therefore, influence the results on the client, we can explore the ways to maximize the relationship between co-therapists and begin to appreciate the complexity of the process. In the following sections, we will outline some specific methods for developing the co-therapy relationship.

Maximizing the Co-therapy Relationship

As we have mentioned, most of what we know about co-therapy comes from the group work literature. One particularly fertile area is the idea that the co-therapy relationship progresses through predictable stages of development, similar to that of a group (Berg, Landreth, & Fall, 2018; Fall & Wejnert, 2005; Gallogly & Levine, 1979; Winter, 1976). Paying attention to the stages can provide an excellent method for assessing relationship progress and highlight obstacles that need to be addressed to facilitate flow and growth. For the application to TCC, we will use the stages outlined by Tuckman and Jensen (1977) and applied to co-leadership by Fall and Wejnert (2005).

Forming

In this beginning phase, the co-leader team is getting to know one another, and this newness produces anxiety. "Will we be able to work together?", "Will the other person like me?", "Will I like them?" are the types of questions that may come up as the relationship begins. Even if the team has worked together before, each new client produces a unique experience. The key thing to remember is that anxiety is normal! Do not avoid it and use it as a motivator to get to know one another and deepen the relationship. This process will take time and effort on each counselor to make it work, much like any other relationship one might create.

In the TCC model, you will be working with the couple in individual counseling at the beginning of the process; forming of the relationship will largely be apart from the clients, which is different from group counseling where the group members are a witness to the developing counselor relationship. In some ways, there are advantages to being able to work on the relationship out of sight, as it gives the co-therapy team opportunities to deepen the connection and not have the clients pry about relationship struggles that will occur. However, this situation may also cause the counselors to ignore the relationship as it is not urgent. Consider this one experience:

My first time working with a co-therapist and trying out the TCC model, we didn't really meet or talk about our relationship until it was time to meet as a foursome—we just didn't think it was important until the joint sessions started. To be honest, it was very awkward walking into that first meeting and realizing we weren't on the same page. I now know that we were trying to get to know one another as we were trying to help the clients. It was awkward and a bit of a mess. We could have saved ourselves and our clients some frustration by realizing that our relationship began the moment we agreed to treat the couple.

As you learn about the TCC model you will see why the relationship, even at this stage, is important. Keep in mind that you will be working with high conflict couples. The rationale for moving the clients into individual counseling prior to couple's sessions mainly rests on the belief that the couple's individual issues and methods for working together as a couple are too maladaptive for one counselor in the traditional couple's mode. Meeting with these clients individually first creates rapport and allows each client to have a safe space to process how their individual issues impact the relationship. These individual sessions will be intense, and each counselor will be charged with balancing the relationship with the client and the relationship with the co-therapy partner. As you can see, paying attention to the co-therapy relationship and attending to it even during the initial stages of the individual sessions, is vital to the co-therapy team and the work with the clients. Having a foundational understanding of the need to focus on the relationship is a good place to start, as the complexity of how to use it within the TCC model will be more apparent as we move through the book.

To enhance the co-therapy relationship in the Forming Stage and increase the probability of a smooth transition into the next phase, co-therapists are encouraged to do the following:

1   Expect anxiety and be aware that this is a normal part of the pilot stages of development. The presence of anxiety does not mean you are an inferior professional. In fact, it only means you are a normal human being reacting to new and exciting opportunities. It is normal for the Forming Stage to be characterized by awkwardness and superficial content. The co-therapists are getting to know each other, so trust and vulnerability are low.

2   Arrange pre- and post-session time to talk with your co-therapist. This time demonstrates a commitment to the relationship and provides a vital opportunity to work on the relationship and process what is going on with the couple. Avoidance of this activity can indicate a disconnect in the relationship, and continuous neglect of the relationship increases the probability of negative consequences for the clients. Meet regularly, even if it is uncomfortable, and might seem unproductive. Use the time to talk about client dynamics, but also spend some time talking about self and getting to know each other.

3   If this is the first time the team has worked together, considering supervision to process the discussion might be helpful. Having an objective person who is also knowledgeable about the importance of the co-therapy relationship can be a powerful catalyst for the developing relationship. The use of supervision in the TCC approach is explored more in-depth in Chapter 7.

Storming

As the co-therapists get to know one another and begin to develop a sense of how each person's identity is integrated and reflected within the team, deeper levels of work begin to emerge. Through session work and outside session processing, each co-therapist should be experiencing a greater knowledge of self and the other co-therapist, both professionally and personally. As depth increases, the need to "play nice" is replaced by the desire to "be real." As Haigh and Kell (1950) noted, "It is often only in the therapeutic relationship with the client that the problems existing between the two therapists become real and apparent. Each is almost forced to become more aware of his strengths and weaknesses as well as learning about each other as therapists" (p. 660). In relationships, this is a positive sign as both parties are no longer afraid of the relationship blowing apart but are willing to risk taking the communication to a deeper level. Roller and Nelson (1991) highlighted five issues that typically contribute to co-therapy conflict and the experience of these issues provide opportunities to practice and demonstrate healthy resolution to the occurrences:

1   Competition: As the relationship develops, it is normal for the co-therapists to try to find their place in the co-therapy-client matrix. When co-therapists vie for control significance within the dyad, these attempts typically get played out in the consultations and in the sessions with the clients. This can often lead to the forming of subgroups within the tandem sessions, as counselors vie to be the "most liked" or "most insightful."
2   Countertransference: Co-therapists' reactions to client dynamics are acted out either in the co-therapy team or with clients. TCC holds these responses to be potentially useful if they are identified and processed in a helpful way, considering both client and co-therapy relationship patterns. Unfortunately, when the relationship is not a focus of the treatment, these issues are often overlooked or ignored.
3   Confusion and lack of communication: Co-therapists who are not openly monitoring and developing the co-therapy relationship have an increased likelihood of dysfunctional communication patterns within that group. Even when paying attention to the relationship, communication errors will occur. It is in those moments, that the co-therapists can identify the disconnect and provide clarity through an open discussion of disagreements and conflict.
4   Incongruence between co-therapists: Differences are expected to exist between two people. In the Storming Stage, the co-therapy relationship has developed enough trust to address the conflict that comes from differences that begin to emerge. Healthy co-therapy

teams will address the conflict that arises from the differences and work through them, making them serviceable for the work. Ineffective co-therapy dyads will become rigid, asserting a level of "rightness" and "wrongness" to one another. This disconnect produces elevated levels of chaos within the relationship and bleeds over into the client dynamics.

5   Co-dependency between co-therapists: As anxiety and conflict intensifies in the co-therapy relationship, one way to manage it is to regress back into the relative superficial safety of the Forming Stage. Another maladaptive method would be to cling onto each other and view the clients as the enemy. Either approach minimizes the potency of the co-therapy relationship by creating obstacles to growth. In the Storming Stage, the co-therapist must see the emerging conflict, both within the co-therapy relationship and within the clients, as a potential for change.

Anticipating these issues and having the courage to work through them will go a long way for developing the skills necessary for a successful partnership. These issues are best identified and explored within the consultation and supervision process that is discussed in detail in Chapter 7.

To test the relationship's durability, the conflict must be experienced and resolved. If the conflict is avoided, the relationship will stagnate. Even worse, the couple will experience the co-therapists' lack of comfort with conflict and will be unable to handle conflict as a couple, paralyzing the work. If the co-therapists are willing to experience conflict but handle it poorly (fight and demean each other in session), the couple will feel an enormous amount of anxiety regarding conflict and either avoid it or replicate the attacking behavior of the counselors and neither is productive for the couple's growth.

It is typical for conflict to begin even before you meet as a foursome. As each counselor works with their client, rapport deepens. The issues and perspectives of each client are being understood, validates, challenged, and explored in depth. It is normal for each counselor to believe in the reality of the client, which varies between the elements of a high conflict couple. As a result, the counselors find themselves connected to parts of the couple's reality in very disparate ways. When the co-therapy team processes this interaction, it is normal for these differences to produce conflict, in much the same ways they produce conflict in the couple. For example:

Counselor A: I was meeting with Susan today. She was really upset about something that happened over the weekend. There had been another mix up in communication and that led to a big fight. For her part, she felt blamed and as a result, she escalated by yelling and demeaning Louis.

Counselor B: Yeah, Louis was pretty mad. He felt like she was dumping it all on him.

Counselor A: Hmm, yeah. What was his part of the pattern?

Counselor B: Not sure about that with this situation. It seemed like it was Susan going off the rails on this one.

Notice how the counselors each drift into their client's perspective and begin to blame the other. This will produce tension in the co-therapy relationship; effective co-leaders will notice the tension and reflect, using it to better understand the clients.

Once the treatment moves to combined sessions, conflict management, and the modeling of healthy conflict, become a potential powerful growth tool. Clients will have the opportunity to process their own conflict in separate ways and, more importantly, allows clients to learn as they witness the co-therapists manage their own conflict as the session progresses.

To increase the probability of transitioning into the next stage, co-therapists are encouraged to focus on the following:

- Understand that the experience of conflict is a normal and necessary part of relationship development. Healthy relationships do not have an absence of conflict, so eradicating conflict should not be the goal of co-therapy nor the couple's. Instead, healthy relationships manage conflict in productive ways. Explore your own gut reaction to the word "conflict." What does it mean to you? Explore past relationships to get a sense of how you handle conflict and consider how those patterns might manifest in the co-therapist relationship and in the group. Talk about these personal insights with your co-therapist.

- Pre- and post-session meetings with your co-therapist are vital during this stage. If one or both of you manage conflict through avoidance, you may notice a tendency to cancel these meetings because "I am too busy." Use these indications as red flags and take time to reinvest in the relationship. It is in these meetings that you can openly discuss your own insights into conflict and collaborate on how it will be processed with the couple. Make sure you are attending to how conflict is emerging and being dealt with in both the co-therapist relationship and in the couple's work.

- Ideally, co-therapy teams have access to a supervisor to help process the conflict that emerges as a normal part of the relationship development. This conflict, along with the patterns identified by the clients, will create a complex confluence of issues that might be difficult for co-therapy dyads to handle on their own. Chapter 7 will explore the intersection between co-therapy consultation and supervision to maximize the potential of TCC.

Norming and Performing Stages

As the co-therapy team moves into the Norming and Performing Stages, the team is building on the patterns that have formed over the previous stages. In general, the relationship has moved from a superficial knowledge of each other to a deeper understanding of professional and personal selves. The conflict has been experienced and methods of healthy resolution of emerging conflict have been established, practiced, and refined in the next two stages. As one counselor expressed:

As I worked with Molly, I got more comfortable learning about myself as I also learned about her. We found it important to talk about personal as well as professional things, so we really began to have a better sense of who we are and where we were coming from ther-apeutically. It made it easier to be vulnerable with her when the couple's work becomes more complicated. I remember saying to her at one point, 'I feel so lost. I don't think I know what I'm doing here.' I don't think I would have been able to do that if we hadn't spent time really developing a close working relationship. Instead of being guarded, we were able to share these feelings, either in actual sessions with the clients or our session debriefings. Once we established the cohesion, we were able to really talk about anything and always ask, 'So how are we going to use this with the couple?' It was an exciting layer to the work!

In this stage, the co-therapy team will be engaged in deeper exploration and understanding of both client and co-therapy dynamics. The transition from Norming and Performing is determined by how ingrained the healthy patterns become; with Norming being characterized by early pattern setting and Performing by more established patterns. As the relationship emerges from conflict resolution at the end of the Storming Stage, the team gets better at processing conflict (inside and outside of the session), is comfortable with the unique identities of each co-therapist, minimizes power struggle, and processes them openly as they occur. In this stage, each co-therapist is committed and invested in the growth and success of the other, which may come through support, encouragement, confrontation, or other aspects of feedback.

It is important to note that the assessments can be taken during the consultation sessions, client sessions, or within supervision, if available. Norming and Performing is about the maintenance of the momentum and deepening of the work with the co-therapy relationship and the client sessions. It is easy during these stages for counselors and clients to feel stagnant—like the momentum has reached a plateau. This feeling of stagnation is normal, and the key is to remember that the relationship is the most effective place to process these emotions and work together to work through any true obstacles and move forward. The following dialogue illustrates this type of exploration between co-therapists.

> Finn: Well, things seem to be going fairly well in the joint sessions. I think both clients are doing a wonderful job focusing on ways to improve the relationship and are providing open and honest feedback to one another.
>
> Lucio: I agree. I thought you did an impressive job last week tying together the two themes of respect and trust. That was new to them, but it added a depth to our work.

Finn: Thanks. I liked how we modeled some of that in session as we were working through the rougher parts.

Lucio: Yeah .... hmmm ... I don't know what else to talk about. I should be happy that things are going well, and we aren't struggling through the crisis du jour, right?

Finn: Yes, I think we are at that point in the counseling where the couple is getting skilled at integrating and using the insights uncovered in our work with them.

Lucio: Yes, it's a good feeling, but I am also feeling a bit restless. When I think about our relationship, I am also excited about the work we have done together, but I think I can be caught between "Is this all there is?" and waiting for the next shoe to drop.

Finn: I think that must be how the clients are feeling too, like, "Is this change for real?" and "Is there any more to be done?". As for us, I agree that I am excited about the progress we have made within the relationship and there is a difference between being *dissatisfied* or restless and *anticipating* growth or restlessness. I'm more of the second one.

Lucio: I see what you mean, and I am there too. It would be bad if the anticipation were perceived as dissatisfaction. We might mention that in the session and see where the clients are in this process.

In this example, the co-therapists openly discuss their feelings about the relationship and the counseling sessions. Their knowledge of the stages of development and their willingness to use the co-therapy relationship as a processing tool facilitates a powerful conceptualization of their feelings and potential impact of their clients. This stage continues until the clients have reached their goals, and the work ends, which moves everyone into the termination stage.

Adjourning/Termination

Termination is the last stage in the relationship, characterized by bringing closure to the experience. With termination processing, the keyword is "balance." When termination is ignored, the effect on the relationship and on the couple's work can be harmful, as the couple may sense that termination is too intense to be processed and should be avoided. Some co-therapists may feel it is unnecessary to process termination issues because they are going to work with each other in the future or are currently working with other couples in TCC. Despite the continuation of the relationship, it is important to be aware that this chapter of this relationship is ending. The team is recognizing that the part of the relationship that was defined by the work with this couple is concluding and deserves to be processed.

We will address issues of termination later in the book, but it is important for now to understand that how you end the counseling experience is just as important as how you begin the work. In the context of co-therapy, it is helpful to be aware of the role that termination plays in the developing co-therapy relationship. In general, co-therapy teams can keep the following in mind as they move toward a termination:

1   Use some time to process and share each other's patterns of saying goodbye. If you tend to avoid goodbyes, then you will tend to do the same within the co-therapy experience. Regardless of the pattern, you have an opportunity to use the co-therapy relationship to experiment with healthier ways of ending relationships.
2   Anxiety at this stage is normal! In fact, each stage of development has its own flavor of anxiety that is inherent within the process. When the anxiety surfaces, make note of it and use that awareness as the foundation of a dialogue about the end of this experience.
3   If you do a decent job with the first two points, then make sure you carve out some time to bring closure to the experience. Many co-therapy teams end with some form of ritual activity and processing, which is appropriate and provides an enjoyable way to end the experience and process any leftover thoughts or feelings about the work or each other.

Utilizing Reflection and Mindfulness in Co-therapy

At this point in the chapter, hopefully, you are aware of the importance of the co-therapy relationship and understand how that relationship might develop over the course of time. While later chapters in this book will give detailed examples of how to weave the relationship dynamics into the TCC process, a few general ways to work on the co-therapy relationship might be helpful here. Because of the emphasis on awareness and open communication, reflection and mindfulness are appropriate areas of focus for developing co-therapy teams. Once again, while these applications were developed with group co-leadership in mind, the concepts are easily adapted to couples' co-therapy work.

Reflective practice in co-therapy is characterized by counselors who routinely and deliberately process how the relationship impacts the counseling, along with and each counselor's own perception of self, the other leader, each client, and the couple as a whole (Okech & Kline 2005). Okech (2008) applied this process of reflective practice to group co-leadership and, along with other researchers, noted the benefits of those co-leader teams that engaged in reflective practice versus those who did not consider the impact of the relationship (Miller 2005; Okech & Kline 2005).

The structure of the reflective process provides a pathway for the seeming complexity of the developing co-therapy relationship. As Okech (2008, p. 239) observed, dedicating time to the process allows each leader to "simultaneously engage in intrapersonal and inter-personal processes, develop insights, which in turn inform their choices on how to engage with each other and group members to promote group member and group objectives." Within this structure, each counselor is encouraged to not only introspect about internal concerns and perceptions but also provides a way to communicate those internal processes to the other counselor and receive feedback.

As an adjunct to the reflective process, the skills and attitudes related to mindfulness can be a helpful way to enact the reflection and con-versations between co-therapists. According to Fulton and Fall (2016), "Mindfulness-based training and interventions have been shown to help individuals attend to sensations, cognitions, and emotions—both po-sitive and negative—with open, non-reactive, non-judging, present-moment awareness (Baer, 2003; Cardaciotto, Herbert, Forman, Moitra, & Farrow, 2008). Thus, mindfulness practice may support reflective practice" (p. X). In integrating mindfulness practice and the reflective process, each step in the structure can be facilitated using mindfulness as a catalyst for promoting greater awareness within the co-therapy team.

For example, during the co-therapist consultation meetings, the co-therapy team could engage in activities associated with the optimal presence. According to Morgan and Morgan (2013), optimal presence is the integration of the factors of awakening which include investigation, joy, energy, tranquility, concentration, and equanimity. Co-therapists can use pre- and post-session meetings to help each other focus on the relationship using these factors. Examples include:

- Investigation: focus on the relationship now; try to understand the client better; try to understand the co-therapy relationship in a deeper way.
- Joy: create a genuine interest in being in the moment and connecting with your partner; generate anticipation of the work with the client and your partner.
- Energy: focus on present anxiety and moving it to a balanced place; explore anxiety operating internally, between co-therapists and between therapist and client.
- Tranquility: focus on acceptance of what is occurring at the moment; as you focus internally, try not to become distracted by the work that may happen in the next hour or by what is happening with your partner. As you direct your attention to the relationship, allow each other to concentrate on the present.
- Concentration: focus on the moment, which includes your body, your breathing, your feelings; as you explore with your partner, stay on topic, and bring distractions into the dialogue.
- Equanimity: this one seems a little vague, but it is the force that pulls each person toward productive elements of the dialogue or experience; co-therapist teams can provide greater awareness by sharing what they perceive or feel as important or interesting with the work with the couple or co-therapy relationship.

While this is just one example of how mindfulness and reflective practice can intersect and be used to develop the co-therapy relationship, we realize that a comprehensive exploration of this process is beyond the scope of this book. We offer this introduction to begin to think about how one might explore and improve the relationship—a way to attend to the relationship in a manner that honors the work involved. In short, we understand that saying, "You need to focus on the co-therapy relationship" is not enough direction to make the relationship a healthy one. In later chapters, we will revisit some of these ideas and provide examples of critical incidents in the co-therapy relationship and different opportunities to focus on the relationship and integrate it into the couple's work. If interested, you can read more about mindfulness practice by consulting Germer, Siegel, and Fulton (2013) or Didonna (2009). Also, Fulton and Fall (2017) outlined how mindfulness could be used across developmental group stages to participate in reflective practice and enhance the co-leader relationship bond.

How to Choose a Co-therapist

Finding a good partner in anything is difficult. When one begins to think of co-therapy as a relationship, the importance of choosing someone who "clicks" with you becomes even more crucial. A good place to begin this discussion is at the top: knowing what factors are associated with successful co-therapy teams. Roller and Neslon's (1991, p. 75) research produced the following six success factors, listed in order of importance:

1 Complementary balance of therapist skills: While a set of TCC-related skills is in Table 7.1, these skills are set as a basic level to maximize the TCC potential. When picking a good co-therapist, start with a comprehensive assessment of your skills as a counselor. A thorough inventory will produce aspects of ease and perceived excellence, as well as elements that might require learning or growth. When seeking a co-therapist, find another person who is not only willing to conduct a similar self-inventory, but also one that has different strengths and weaknesses from your own. For example, if you are good at working with the cognitive aspects of client material but struggle with intense emotions, then find a partner who is strong in connecting on an affective level. This type of pairing will provide depth to your collective skillset.

2   Compatibility of the therapist's theoretical viewpoints: It is not necessary for co-therapists to share the same theory of practice, but it is important that each have congruent philosophical underpinnings. To discern the core beliefs of a theory, one does not look at the techniques but at the philosophy that provides the roots of the approach. Much in the way we discussed philosophy in Chapter 3, every theory has philosophical assumptions about how people develop, struggle, and change. While some theories have considerable overlap with one another, some create contradictions that, when practiced together, would produce confusion in the co-therapy approach and have negative outcomes for the clients. For example, it might be easy for any theory that has an existential, constructivist, or phenomenological base to work with another that shares that foundation, while it would be very difficult for that same family of theories to work with one that holds a more deterministic philosophy. While it is beyond the scope of this book to provide a full comparison and contrast of all the available theories, each practitioner should be able to explain their own theory of practice. For s survey of the major theories, along with the philosophical underpinnings of each, consult Fall, Holden, and Marquis (2017).

3   Openness in communication: For co-therapy to work to its full potential, the co-therapists must talk to one another. It is through open communication that growth occurs in the co-therapy team and in the couple's sessions. When we speak of "openness," what we are really referring to is the counselor's willingness to disclose aspects of self, perceptions about the clients, and feelings and thoughts regarding the other counselor and the co-therapy relationship. Without honest discourse, co-therapy is lacking in its power. According to Roller and Nelson (1991) this communication occurs at four main levels: in pre-session consultations; during the session; in post-session consultations; and sharing elements of personal life that might impact the counseling. We would add supervision as an additional helpful level. In utilizing all the levels, the co-therapy dyad has the most opportunity to relationally evolve and integrate aspects of the relationship into the treatment of the couple.

4   Equality of participation: In healthy co-therapy teams, both partners
will share the responsibility of facilitation during the joint sessions.
While in the beginning, co-therapists may try to apply structure to
this by assigning tasks within the sessions. For example, one person
may handle opening the session and the other, closing; process
observation for one, content remarks for the other. While this might
work in group counseling or other approaches other than TCC, we
find that this sort of structure is unnecessary. As you will learn, TCC
uses individual sessions at the beginning of the counseling process,
which allows time for both client and counselor to establish a
meaningful rapport and a feeling of connection and significance that
they carry into the joint sessions. Even with this advantage, it is
important for co-therapy dyads to be aware of personal and client
parallel process dynamics that might impact the level of participation.
Through this awareness, the patterns can be discussed with the co-
therapy consultations and utilized in the joint sessions to promote
insight and pathways for change in the couple.

5   Liking each other as people: While it is not absolutely necessary to
like your co-therapist, it certainly is preferable and makes the
process much more enjoyable. Liking someone does not mean an
absence of conflict or disagreement, but it speaks more to how the
conflict is handled. If you like someone, you are more willing to
find a mutual goal and work toward a solution. You are more likely
to give the other person the benefit of the doubt and less likely to
demonize them or move to disconnect. Using the elements of high
conflict discussed in Chapter 2, it is difficult to imagine those
elements existing with a person you genuinely like. If you are
working with a new co-therapist, it may be difficult to know
whether you like them or not, but focusing on the relationship (in
the ways we have discussed so far) provide you with the best
avenue for cultivating a relationship that is enjoyable for you. If you
realize you do not like them, you can always select another partner!

6   Respect: Mutual respect is vital to many of the TCC based co-therapy
skills. Without respect, the co-therapy relationship is vulnerable to
competition among the co-therapists and increases the likelihood of
client exploitation. In relationships where respect is not present, co-
therapists will   jockey   for   attention—undermining   each   other,

modeling poor relationship skills, and paralyzing client progress. In such a toxic relationship, it is better to refer the couple to a new counselor than proceed with the current treatment structure. Respect can be sensed even in the first interview. If your prospective partner is late to your first interview or refuses to meet to discuss the possible pairing, is not interested in getting to know you, does not take your interest with them seriously, or spends an inordinate amount of time focusing on their abilities, then you might be experiencing the seeds of disrespect. It is well within your power to persevere and meet multiple times to see if respect can grow but if the pattern persists, it is better to look elsewhere for a partner before committing to treating a couple.

Similarly, Nelson-Jones (1992, p. 58) offered these practical suggestions for choosing a co-leader:

- Take the time to interview your prospective co-therapist. Many co-therapist teams are created out of convenience. Although that is not a highly effective way to choose a compatible co-therapist, it is the reality of the field. Even if you are assigned to a person, set up a pre-counseling session to discuss the other items on this list.
- Work with people who have theoretical positions like your own. You each need to understand the underlying philosophies that guide and define your change process. As mentioned earlier in this chapter, it is not required that you practice identical theories, but the theories should be philosophically congruent. An effective way to approach this with your prospective co-therapist, beyond asking them their theory of practice, is to share your respective beliefs about how people develop, the origins of maladjustment, and how change occurs.
- Work with people with whom you can have a cooperative and honest relationship. In the beginning, this might be difficult to discern. As noted in the developmental stage discussion, you both will be trying to connect with the other person and be accepted. Try to acknowledge this developmental process and work to openly disclose your way of doing things and your expectations of how counseling will unfold, then hear your co-therapist's reflections. Assess yourself during the interview: How much did you hold back?

- Commit time to work with each other before and after each counseling session. Bridbord and DeLucia-Waack's (2011) research concluded that this was a vital aspect of co-leader satisfaction in groups. In our experience with co-therapy, it is not unusual to spend about 30 minutes prior to the session discussing the themes and related issues that might be pertinent to the upcoming work. After the session, another 30 minutes can be used to debrief and process the day's work. When interviewing potential co-therapists, I (KAF) ask them to look at their weekly schedule on their phone or book. If we are planning on meeting the clients on Tuesday at 4:00, I will say, "Look at your schedule. Can you be free from 3-6 PM on Tuesday?". If the answer is no, then I am doubtful the person is able to put in the time that will be needed to develop the relationship. In our opinion, if you cannot commit to the relationship in the beginning—when everything is exciting and fresh—it is going to be near-impossible to devote time later when the challenging work begins.

In addition to the guidelines above, we would also encourage you to consider attending the supervision of your co-therapy, especially if you are new to the process or are working with a new person. Making supervision a part of the process early increases the chance that you will sidestep any relationship problems and provides the team with an outlet should problems occur. Once you get comfortable with the co-therapy process, you may want to serve as a supervisor or consultant for other co-therapy teams. Doing so helps create a community of co-therapists who value the relationship as a force for therapeutic change. We will discuss this process in more detail in Chapter 7.

Roller and Nelson (1991) constructed a Co-therapy Issues Questionnaire to be used when selecting a co-therapist. All the questions on their inventory are closed-ended, so we have adapted and modified the items for our own work with TCC. Below are some of the key questions one can use to assess the fit of co-therapy options.

1 Describe your therapeutic self.
2 Discuss how you use a confrontation with clients. With co-therapists.

3 Explain how you use here and now processing in co-therapy sessions.

4 Explain how you use historical information in co-therapy sessions.

5 In what ways do you feel competent/confident in your work? In what ways do you struggle?

6 Discuss how you convey acceptance and empathy to your clients.

7 What does co-therapy mean to you?

8 Describe how much time you would like to invest in developing the co-therapy relationship. Outline what you would do with that time.

9 What types of personality dynamics frustrate you? How do you typically deal with these issues?

10 Describe your current intimate relationship. How would you describe the patterns of your relational self?

Does Gender Matter in Co-therapist Selection?

In traditional models of couples therapy, working with a single counselor, the impact of gender rests on the manifestation of that gender on the part of the counselor, the perception of gender from the client's perspective, and how those gender roles play out within the couple relationship. Here are some examples of gender-based struggles a single counselor may confront in couple's work with heterosexual couples (adapted from Ficher & Linsenberg, 1976)

• As rapport is built with an opposite-sex client, the partner feels like the counselor is trying to seduce their partner.

• As rapport is built with same-sex clients, the partner feels like the counselor is relating to their partner because they are the "same." The result is the opposite sex client feels misunderstood and "ganged upon."

• Unhealthy manifestations of stereotypical gender roles emerge in the counseling. A female client is passive and agreeable to a male counselor; a dominant focused male client competes for control with a female counselor.

These examples may seem stereotypical and not reflective of what you might expect from a progressive society, but these examples are common in practice. In fact, as early as 1977, research showed that couples who struggled with rigid marriage roles were more apt to seek counseling than those with more egalitarian views (Rice & Rice, 1977). The point is not that traditional gender roles are bad, but understanding how the roles impact the relationship is an important consideration. This book outlines an approach for high conflict couples and in this population, unhealthy patterns—including extreme gender roles—are even more present.

The dynamics become even more layered when working with transgender or gender-fluid therapists and clients, as those identities become an added opportunity for perceptions to impact the work, both with clients and in the co-therapy pair. The key question, regardless, of co-therapy gender configuration, is not if gender impacts the co-therapy relationship and the work with clients, but how gender interacts within these two aspects of TCC. This important question can be processed throughout the counseling both in the co-therapy discussion as well as with the couple. The consideration of how any element of diversity, race, spirituality, socio-economic status, sexual identity, age, or other facets can be explored through the same lens.

You might be wondering how and when to facilitate this exploration with a co-therapist. We think the discussion will look different depending on the stage of development. Forming Stage teams might have discussions based on how each person identifies. What roles are important to you? The emphasis of this stage is usually on aspects of identity that are comfortable for each member. The team is trying to create a sense of cohesion and belonging so the personal sharing will reflect that goal. Storming Stage relationships can experiment with deeper level conversations and processing differences become important at this stage. As the team becomes more comfortable with each other, more authentic discussions can occur.

Although past research makes some excellent points regarding the possible impact of gender on the co-therapy relationship and how those dynamics may affect clients, there seem to be few definitive conclusions beyond these considerations. What we can conclude is that the quality of the relationship between co-therapists is a key element to consider when selecting and developing a co-therapist relationship. With any gender configuration, co-therapists can be mindful of how the relationships model egalitarian, mutually supportive roles and can be open to discussing these issues, both with each other and with the clients.

Summary

This chapter is designed to illuminate the co-therapy relationship as the clinical rationale for choosing this modality of couples counseling. A model of reflective practice and mindfulness was offered as one means of developing and attending to the relationship. With this knowledge on the importance of the relationship, we can revisit the case at the beginning of the chapter and understand why Blake was so anxious about his co-therapy arrangement. This case exemplifies everything that is wrong, but far too common, in the practice of co-therapy. No planning. No relationship development. No training in co-therapy. Blake, his co-therapist, and their clients were being set up in an environment that has a high probability to be ineffective at a minimum and harmful at the most to the parties involved.

As we move forward in the book, it is essential to keep the co-therapy relationship central to your understanding of how TCC works. The next chapters in the book will contain more detail on the process of TCC and will, at times, primarily focus on the client dynamics, but it is vital to always consider the role the co-therapy relationship is playing in every aspect of the counseling—both in and out of session. We hope that by reading this material, you are somewhat overwhelmed by the amount of time and energy needed to foster a quality co-therapy relationship. Good! We also hope that the overwhelmed feeling is accompanied by excitement about what could happen if you were to participate in such a relationship. In our experience, some of the most personally and professionally fulfilling experiences have been as a part of a healthy co-therapy relationship. We feel it is worth the effort! To end this chapter, we close with a quote from Roller and Nelson (1991), "Co-therapy teams are developed. They do not spring fully formed into the therapeutic milieu. Time is needed. Concentration and hard work and listening are required… Co-therapists must know more than therapists, and more is required of them than of solo therapists" (p. 41).

References

Baer, R. A. (2003). Mindfulness training as a clinical intervention: A conceptual and empirical review. *Clinical Psychology: Science and Practice*, *10*(1), 125–143.

Berg, R. C., Landreth, G. L., & Fall, K. A. (2018). *Group counseling: Concepts and procedures* (6th ed.). New York: Routledge.

Bridbord, K., & DeLucia-Waack, J. (2011). Personality, leadership style and theoretical orientation as predictors of group co-leadership satisfaction. *The Journal for Specialists in Group Work, 36*(3), 202–221.

Cardaciotto, L., Herbert, J. D., Forman, E. M., Moitra, E., & Farrow, V. (2008). The assessment of present-moment awareness and acceptance: The Philadelphia Mindfulness Scale. *Assessment, 15*(2), 204–223.

Didonna, F. (2009). *Clinical handbook of mindfulness.* New York: Springer.

Ellickson, J. L., & Seals, T. (1986). Gender and intimacy: Cotherapy with a premarital couple. *Psychotherapy: Theory, Research, Practice, Training, 23*(2), 274–282.

Fall, K. A., Holden, J. M., & Marquis, A. C. (2017). *Theoretical models of counseling and psychotherapy* (3rd ed.). New York: Routledge.

Fall, K. A., & Menendez, M. (2002). Seventy years of co-leadership: Where are we now? *Texas Counseling Association Journal, 30*, 24–33.

Fall, K. A., & Wejnert, T. J. (2005). Co-leader stages of development: An application of Tuckman and Jensen (1977). *Journal for Specialists in Group Work, 30*(4), 309–327.

Ficher, I. V., & Linsenberg, M. (1976). Problems confronting the female therapist doing couple therapy. *Journal of Marital and Family Therapy, 2*(2), 331–340.

Fulton, C., & Fall, K. A. (2016). Mindfulness as a mechanism for developing the co-leader relationship. *Groupwork, 25*(1), 6–24.

Germer, C. K., Siegel, R. D., & Fulton, P. R. (2013). In C. K. Germer, R. D. Siegel & P. R. Fulton (Eds.), *Mindfulness and psychotherapy* (2nd ed.). New York, NY: Guilford Press.

Gallogly, V., & Levine, B. (1979). Co-therapy. In B. Levine (Ed.), *Group psychotherapy: Practice and development* (pp. 296–305). Prospect Heights, IL: Waveland.

Haigh, G., & Kell, B. L. (1950). Multiple therapy as a method for training and research in psychotherapy. *The Journal of Abnormal and Social Psychology, 45*(4), 659–666.

Haley, J. (1996). *Learning and teaching therapy.* New York: Guilford.

Hendrix, C.C., Fournier, D.G., & Briggs, K. (2001). Impact of co-therapy teams on client outcomes and therapist training in marriage and family therapy. *Contemporary Family Therapy, 23*(1), 63–82.

McMahon, N., & Links, P. S. (1984). Cotherapy: The need for positive pairing. *Canadian Journal of Psychiatry, 29,* 385–389.

Mehlman, S. K., Baucom, D. H., & Anderson, D. (1983). Effectiveness of cotherapists versus single therapists and immediate versus delayed treatment in behavioral marital therapy. *Journal of Consulting and Clinical Psychology, 51*(2), 258–266.

Miller, S. (2005). What it's like being the "holder of the space": A narrative on working with reflective practice in groups. *Reflective Practice, 6,* 367–377.

Morgan, W. D., & Morgan, S. T. (2013). Cultivating attention and empathy. In C. K. Germer, R. D. Siegel & P. R. Fulton (Eds), *Mindfulness and psychotherapy* (pp. 73–90). New York: Guilford.

Nelson-Jones, R. (1992). *Group leadership: A training approach.* Belmont, CA: Brooks Cole.

Okech, J. A. (2008). Reflective practice in group-co-leadership. *Journal for Specialists in Group Work, 33*(3), 236–253.

Okech, J. E. A., & Kline, W. B. (2005). A qualitative exploration of group co-leader relationships. *The Journal for Specialists in Group Work, 30*(2), 173–190.

Rice, D. G., & Rice, J. (1977). Non-sexist 'martital' therapy. *Journal of Marital and Family Therapy, 3*(1), 3–10.

Roller, B., & Nelson, V. (1991). *The art of co-therapy.* New York: Guilford.

Tuckman, B. W., & Jensen, M. C. (1977). Stages of small group development revisited. *Group and Organizational Studies, 2*(4), 419–427.

Winter, S. K. (1976). Developmental stages in the roles and concerns of group co-leaders. *Small Group Behavior, 7*(3), 349–362.

5

TANDEM COUPLES COUNSELING PROTOCOL

The previous chapters have attempted to provide the foundation for the Tandem Couples Counseling (TCC) approach. Most notably, TCC was developed to address high conflict couples—couples for whom more traditional forms of counseling had been ineffective. We rely on the assessment of the high conflict, along with the unique synthesis of co-therapy literature largely drawn from the field of group counseling, to provide these clients with a different way of working with their relationship patterns. This chapter will provide an outline of the process of TCC. To help illuminate the process, we will use the case of Stan and Lacy. Each step of the process will be explored, and the client and co-therapy dynamics explained. An overview of the general process can be found in Figure 5.1.

Step One: Initial Contact

Couples enter counseling in several ways. In most cases, the appropriateness for TCC is not apparent during the first phone call, so for

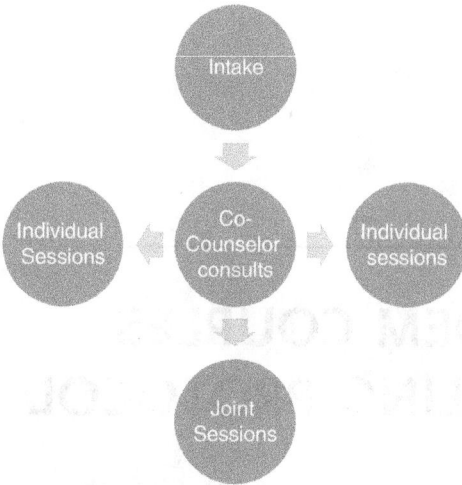

Figure 5.1 Tandem Couples Counseling Process.

deciding about TCC, the importance is not much on how clients come into counseling, but what to do once they get there. Stan and Lacy enter counseling the way many couples do—with a phone call—in this case, by Lacy. We are going to give a few examples of this form of the first contact because how a client enters counseling can give the counselor different information about the patterns of the relationship and the couple's approach to the problem.

First Contact Example #1

Lacy:	Hello, I am interested in couples counseling.
Dr. Levitov:	Ok, that sounds good. Tell me a little about what you are looking to change.
Lacy:	Well, it's nothing that serious. We have communication problems.
Dr. Levitov:	You and your partner are having difficulty talking to one another and you would like counseling to help.

Lacy:	Pretty much. We would like to get in as soon as possible.
Dr. Levitov:	Ok, it looks like I have availability next Thursday evening.
Lacy:	Hmm... is there any way we can get in sooner than that? We really need the help.
Dr. Levitov:	It sounds like you are really motivated. It's Friday evening and I don't see clients on the weekends. In looking at my schedule, Thursday is my next opening and I have that time open consistently, so we will be able to meet at that time weekly if that works for you.
Lacy:	Is there any way you could make an exception and see us on Saturday?
Dr. Levitov:	Unfortunately, no. Will Thursday at 6:00 work? If that doesn't work for you, I would be happy to provide some names of counselors who work on the weekends.
Lacy:	I guess that will work. I don't want to go through the hassle of trying to call someone else. If something earlier opens, let us know. Otherwise, we will see you on Thursday.

This first contact may seem commonplace and in fact, you may have had similar conversations with prospective clients, but there are some interesting therapeutic elements even in this trivial introduction. Paying attention to the first contact, you will be surprised at the wealth of information being shared. What are some of the elements that provide clues about possible client issues and patterns? First, it's standard for couples to state "communication problems" as the presenting problem. While almost all couples can improve their communication, that is usually not the most pressing issue and is usually a safe area of the relationship.

Next, you might notice the subtle boundary testing that occurs regarding the session appointment. The client creates a sense of urgency by pressing to be seen sooner than the counselor offers. When the counselor restates the boundary, the client tests the boundary by asking for special accommodation—in this case, asking the counselor to meet on weekends. In working with clients, boundaries are important as they contribute to a sense of consistency, stability, and safety necessary to the counseling atmosphere. With high conflict couples, firm boundaries are even more important, as the counselor can expect the client to bring a large amount of chaos with them into the therapeutic encounter. With the first contact, you might not know whether the couple is high conflict or not, but regardless, setting firm boundaries will provide important norms for the developing relationship between client and counselor.

First Contact Example #2

Lacy:	Hello, I am interested in couples counseling.
Dr. Levitov:	Ok, that sounds good. Tell me a little about what you are looking to change.
Lacy:	Well, it's nothing that serious. We have communication problems.
Dr. Levitov:	You and your partner are having difficulty talking to one another and you would like counseling to help.
Lacy:	Pretty much. We would like to get in as soon as possible.
Dr. Levitov:	Ok, it looks like I have availability next Thursday evening.
Lacy:	Oh, can we come on Monday? After that, we are leaving for vacation for three weeks and were hoping to get in before that.
Dr. Levitov:	Actually, it would be better to begin after your vacation. Why don't we set something up for the Thursday of your return?
Lacy:	(sighs) I guess that will work.

In this example, we illustrate the common occurrence for couples to decide to come in right before they will not be available for a period, in this case, a vacation. We conceptualize this as a way for the couple to "participate without commitment", which means the couple can say they are working on the problem (initiating counseling) but then escaping by failing to commit to the long process. The initial contact is about orienting the clients to the norms of counseling, so delaying the start of counseling until the commitment can be made communicates the importance of consistency moving forward. Overall, regardless of the content of the first contact, we are stressing the importance of paying attention to the process of the exchange and use that information to begin to form tentative hypotheses about the relational patterns.

Step Two: Intake and Assessment

After getting the couple in the door, we see the first 1–4 sessions as an assessment period with any clients—couple or individual. So, at this stage, the decision for traditional or TCC has not been made. We are gathering information and building rapport with the clients. Levitov and Fall (2019) outline the purpose of these initial sessions and the elements are useful within this protocol:

1   Gather information about the client
2   Orient the client to the process of counseling
3   Formulate tentative goals
4   Test the alliance

Couples may be offered TCC as a treatment option at various points in their effort to pursue counseling. The elements of a high conflict couple, as discussed in Chapter 2, provide the assessment for the appropriateness of offering TCC as a treatment option. It is when these elements begin to surface in the beginning sessions, that the counselor may begin to consider the TCC approach. Most often, such couples are identified during a standard intake evaluation process where they are seen first as a couple. As the counselor begins to detect the elements of high conflict in the couple's history, the counselor also pays attention to how those dynamics are impacting the current therapeutic relationship. It is based on these two strands of evidence (history and immediacy), that the decision to move to individual intakes for further assessment can be made. This standard, four-session intake process is quite common.

When couples' issues meet the criteria for TCC, the option is explained and offered as one treatment pathway at the fourth meeting.

We also receive referrals from other mental health practitioners who specifically request TCC for their clients, and some clients are offered TCC as a protocol change after traditional efforts fail to produce the desired results. In all cases, the rationale for suggesting a change in treatment options is carefully explained. Except for compelling reasons against a traditional approach (e.g., domestic violence), clients make the choice after discussing the option with their partner. They are encouraged to take their time in deciding so they will often leave the fourth session with a plan to talk over the choice and contact us once they decide.

When done thoroughly and properly, the intake process usually provides sufficient information about the couple's relationship history, the family of origin issues, and current concerns for an assessment of the couple's suitability for TCC. The history of potential domestic violence makes TCC an obvious and immediate alternative. Other factors do not alone constitute the recommendation, though couples who have a history of failed attempts or who experience difficulties on several of the other factors are often encouraged to consider TCC as an option.

Couples and counselors cooperate in determining how well TCC meets their needs. Many couples experienced previous failed attempts at therapy, so the offer of a uniquely different protocol often sparks interest and hopefulness. They seem buoyed by such an unusual way to begin therapy—each meeting with their own counselor. The idea of eventually meeting as a foursome calms them because they sense an advocate with them when they begin the couple's component of the counseling. They seem to sense that the protocol not only produces less anxiety but also contains the anxiety that surfaces. We find it remarkable that explaining simple structural changes affects the couple so quickly.

Here is what was uncovered in the first session with Stan and Lacy:

Stan is 45 and Lacy is 40. They have been married for 18 years and have two daughters, aged 11 and 15. Stan works in sales for a company owned by his father-in-law. Lacy describes herself as a "stay-at-home mom who has an active social life". They have come in for counseling because they each believe that their relationship has so seriously deteriorated that they are, for the first time, considering separating.

They report little success with past attempts with counseling. They first saw a counselor who some years earlier treated Lacy's parents. While her parents did not return to this counselor, they did become—and have remained—social friends. Despite the counselor's assurances, Stan worried his personal information would get back to his "boss," Lacy's father. Lacy thought Stan's fears were "childish and ridiculous". They next tried couples counseling three years ago but left after only a few sessions. For the second attempt, Stan chose the counselor. Lacy described her as "a blonde bimbo who was only interested in flirting with Stan and taking his side on every issue." Stan feels Lacy just can't tolerate anyone paying him the slightest amount of attention, "even though [she] ignore[s] me most of the time." Most recently, they saw a couple's counselor about a year ago, but soon quit after two sessions. Stan said the counselor "just stared at them the entire time," but Lacy believed that the counselor "just wasn't interested in working with us".

The couple's premarital histories offered many clues to the source of their difficulty: Lacy's parents were married at an early age. Her mom remained home to raise her family, while her father worked long hours and eventually became the sole owner of a large manufacturing company. She describes her childhood as "lonely." Her dad, a self-proclaimed "workaholic," rarely saw her and mom—mostly unavailable due to alcohol dependence. She sees mom as "weak" and dad as "very controlling". Absentee parents prompted Lacy to develop a close relationship with her older sister. She continues to find comfort in that relationship. She also credits her faith in the Roman Catholic Church as another source of strength in her life.

Stan's family, in his words, was a "disaster." Stan is an only child. His father committed suicide when Stan was eight years old, but Stan denies knowing why. Stan's mother remarried four times and recently died from a heart attack. Stan reports that he learned nothing about relationships from his parents, but states, "I must be a natural because I have been married to the same woman forever".

Lacy's perspective of the presenting problem: "We don't communicate; we fight about everything. He always must be right and won't listen to a word I say. He is inconsistent with the children. He is selfish and a poor lover."

Stan's perspective of the problem: "I don't see anything wrong with our marriage. After all, we've been married 18 years. It's 99% perfect. The 1%? She refuses to kiss me."

Elements of High Conflict

By way of a reminder, Chapter 2 contained the following examples of problems that might inhibit effective couples counseling and encourage offering TCC as a more functional alternative to the couple. Our couple meets many of the elements of a high conflict couple.

In Chapter 2, typologies from both Gottman and Silver (1999) and Anderson, Anderson, Palmer, Mutchler, and Baker (2011) were explored as structures for identifying high conflict couples. Applying this, it is easy to see elements of Criticism, Contempt and Defensiveness, and Stonewalling. Criticism in ingrained in their interactions and the way they criticize is reflected in their relational patterns. Stan, in his attempt to avoid conflict, will criticize Lacy's "negativity" to get her to back off and leave him alone; Lacy uses criticism to perturb Stan into action. Contempt is most noticeable in Lacy's communication and perception of Stan. They both report feeling disrespected by the other, but Lacy employs contempt regularly to highlight the dissatisfaction she has with Stan. If contempt is the primary tool of Lacy, Stan is the master of defensiveness and stonewalling. As Lacy takes a more assertive stance, Stan responds by becoming defensive. As Lacy encounters the defenses, she becomes more frustrated and intensifies her criticism and contempt, and Stan counters with stonewalling. This pattern, indicative of high conflict, shuts down opportunities for growth, and make counseling particularly challenging. This next example provides evidence of all four elements in one brief interchange.

Counselor:	Tell me a little bit about what you hope to gain from counseling.
Lacy:	Stan, why don't you start. I would like to hear your answer to this.
Stan:	I don't know. Why do I have to start?
Lacy:	Because I always go first. It's time for you to step up and stop making me do everything.
Stan:	I don't know what to say when you put me on the spot like that? What's the big deal with you going first?
Lacy:	Stop being such a dimwit. Just answer the counselor's question!

Counselor: Yes, everyone will have a chance to answer because I am interested in both perspectives. Lacy, Stan seems pressured by your offer for him to go first, so why don't you go ahead and give your perspective, and then we can hear from him. As we move on in the work, we'll make sure to pay attention to balancing the sharing.

Lacy: Great, another counselor who takes Stan's side.

Counselor: I'm just trying to stay focused on the goal of hearing your story and not getting stuck in the pattern.

Stan: I don't even know how to answer the question, so yeah, you go first.

Lacy: How can you pretend to not know how to answer that question? It's easy, Stan. What do you want to get out of counseling? Why are you here, Stan? Why are you in this relationship, Stan? What's your problem, Stan?

Stan: I don't know what you want me to say.

Assessing Stan and Lacy from Anderson et al.'s (2011) typology of high conflict, we can see evidence of both Clusters I: Pervasive Negative Exchanges and II: Hostile. Insecure, Emotional Environment. For Cluster I, the communication between Stan and Lacy is described by Lacy as a "constant storm fighting". What makes their relationship interesting is that Stan tries to mediate the conflict by ignoring it; however, it is counterproductive. The rigid lockdown into this pattern is what makes the relationship so volatile. You might see this same dynamic in other, less intense relationships, but the communication spiral is looser, which means the intense reactions are more spread out and creates spaces for change. With Stan and Lacy, the spiral is tight, where one intense reaction is stacked right next to the other, with no perceived space for de-escalation. In the exchange below, notice how quickly the negative arises and the paralysis that emerges in the counseling.

Counselor: It sounds like you had a decent weekend. You created some time to spend together and process some of the issues we touched on in the first session.

Lacy: I had to literally threaten him to get him to do it, though.

Stan: I have no idea what you are talking about.

Lacy: You were going to go play basketball with your buddies—you had no intention to spend time with me. I had to make a big scene to get you to spend one freaking hour with me and, even then, you couldn't wait to get away.

Stan: You're crazy.

Counselor: Let's pause for a moment and look at what is happening. I—

Lacy: (interrupts):—I'm crazy?! If I am, it's because you made me that way. How pathetic does a man have to be to not be able to spend one hour with his wife over the weekend? You'd rather hang out with your stupid friends and play. Grow up, Stan. You are an old man, so stop trying to recreate your 20s.

Counselor: Ok, we seem to be getting off track. I was trying to focus on what went right this weekend and—

Stan: —she can't do that; it's not in her genes. She's just like her father and will not be satisfied until she has demeaned everyone in the room. Let me tell you: you aren't so special yourself.

For Cluster II, it should be evident that their relationship is permeated with a constant blanket of hostility and defensiveness. There seems to be no motivation to be vulnerable; their patterns are firmly rooted in the negative elements of Active-Passive (Lacy-Stan) pattern of interaction. As each move to their respective corners, they employ behaviors that reinforce the lack of safety and trust within the relationship. They are also skilled at triangulating others into their conflict. Past participants have included Lacy's father, a few friends, and their children.

We now move to explore the additional elements of high conflict that might be useful to you in assessing your couples and their potential appropriateness for TCC.

Domestic Violence/Abuse

This couple did not endorse a history of domestic violence and abuse, and the initial interview did not unearth the probability in either client.

Severe Psychopathology

While unhappy about their circumstances and discouraged about their future together, they did not report symptoms that could be consistent with more serious psychopathology. Neither reports a history of mental illness nor has received a formal diagnosis. If evidence of a diagnosis emerged during the intake, a psychiatric referral may be considered and discussed with the client. If either client reports a psychiatric history, consent to consult with the psychiatrist or other medical profession could be helpful in learning the context of the previous treatment.

Family of Origin Concerns

Each of the couple disclosed information about their respective legacy to warrant concern. Growing up in a family exposes us to models of relating. Parents, for better or worse, repetitively offer a relationship model. Such lessons persist long after leaving the environment we grew up in. One client beautifully stressed the point when he reflected on how inappropriately he behaved toward his wife. He looked up, clearly feeling some sense of shame, and said, "I just keep using my dad's playbook and my wife deserves better." The insight was even more important because he despised the way his dad treated his mother.

Stan's father passed away when he was only eight years old; his mother remarried four times. When he calls himself a "natural" at relationships he is not far-off if we use his family of origin as criterion. Unfortunately, Stan has little insight on how this blueprint operates in his relationship. This lack of insight leads him to feel confused and is at a greater risk of externalizing and blaming Lacy. Experiencing the loss of both caretakers at such an early age may lead Stan to have a hypersensitivity to abandonment, which could manifest as possessiveness or apathy in relationships due to fear that "everyone eventually leaves, so why bother?"

Lacy identifies a family pattern rich with conflicts. While her parents remained together, their relationship modeled a range of insoluble problems. She possesses clear perspectives on both her parents and expresses a decent amount of insight into how these patterns have impacted her relationships. Unfortunately, the insights did not help her much in her current relationship, and she seems more caught up in the patterns rather than being ready to change. As a result, she actively tries to avoid the pattern she perceives in her mom (weakness and passivity), but begins to feel more like her father (controlling) as she moves away, and she doesn't like that either. This ping-pong effect creates anxiety in Lacy, and she typically copes with it by blaming Stan.

The review of the legacy issues also surfaces several strengths. Most noteworthy, even though each brings such complicated histories to the relationship, they are still together. And they seem to be focused, though not always successfully, on making their children's lives better than those they experienced in their early years. Their struggles testify to how difficult it can be to rewrite the "gamebook" and in doing so, enact significant changes.

History of Disturbed Relationships

Both clients observed relationship problems in their families of origin. The difficulties they experienced in earlier dating relationships echoed the trouble they saw at home. While they never used the term "intimacy" beyond referring to their physical relationship, they seemed to understand that what was missing in their marital relationship seemed to be missing in all their previous relationships and in the relationships that they observed.

While most couples have a history of failed relationships, in high conflict couples, these failures do not produce growth, and typically produces resentment, externalization, and stagnation or paralysis of relationship development. These elements create unique challenges in couple's therapy which contributes to poor treatment outcomes. Lacy and Stan's past relationships have contributed to significant issues that interfere with counseling. The example below illustrates one of these issues, which we call "Competing Reality Syndrome".

Dr. Levitov:	Let's talk about how the couple deals with conflict and disagreement. Give me an example of a recent disagreement and how it was handled.
Stan:	I can't really remember one. I think we tend to do a fairly decent job of dealing with things.
Lacy:	(rolls her eyes) Oh please, we fought on the way here. He didn't want to come—he said that counseling is for losers.
Stan:	I didn't say that.
Lacy:	Stan! We had this fight last night and this morning. You said counselors are fucking losers and why would you pay someone to fix something that isn't broken.
Stan:	I did NOT say that. I have never been to counseling before, so I was asking you if you thought it would help.
Lacy:	You did not even ask that. You said it was bullshit and threatened to fake being sick.
Stan:	I never said that.

In "Competing Reality Syndrome" the clients will have a completely different version of events—so different that all one can learn from their conflict resolution strategy is they move very far apart, making the identification of a mutual goal all but impossible. Whereas all couples will do this to some extent, high conflict couples use it rigidly and consistently, fueling the conflict instead of providing a pathway to remedy it. As noted in Chapter 2, in many cases of high conflict couples, it happens so often that it will happen in a session, but the couple will compete with the counselor's reality as well. Stan and Lacy illustrate this point.

Lacy:	My father gave Stan a job. I'm not sure if Stan is living up to his end of the bargain, which puts a strain on me.
Dr. Levitov:	Tell me more about the strain it puts on you.
Lacy:	I feel like I am responsible for Stan keeping his job and keeping the family afloat. I must be nice to my dad, so he doesn't get fired!

Stan:	That's not true. Everything at work is fine. Your father and I have a fine relationship.
Lacy:	How can you say that? You complain about work all the time.
Stan:	No, I don't. I mean I talk about work stuff, but it's fine.
Dr. Levitov:	Lacy, you mentioned the stress it puts on you to feel you must mediate between your father and Stan. What does that look like?
Lacy:	I never said I had to mediate their disagreements. Why would that be my responsibility?
Dr. Levtiov:	Well, I thought you said you had to be kind to your father to make up for Stan's effort or performance at work.
Lacy:	No, I said that Stan is lucky to have a job and he doesn't show that appreciation to anyone.
Stan:	I show appreciation all the time.
Lacy:	No, you don't.
Dr. Levitov:	So you would like him to be more appreciative.
Lacy:	I never said that. It's not my job to make him appreciate anything. He should do that on his own.
Dr. Levitov:	So you don't want to feel like you are making him appreciate you or your father.
Lacy:	I don't care is he appreciates my father. My father is an asshole.
Stan:	And the problem is, I do show appreciation all the time. She just doesn't see it.

In this example, as well as any of the other aspects of dysfunctional relationship patterns, the expression is more extreme and rigid than with most couples. Addressing these issues with a traditional approach can be very frustrating to all parties.

From a clinical perspective, Stan and Lacy have accomplished the infatuation stage of their relationship but stalled as they tried to transition from infatuation to intimacy. Many couples experience this problem because the transition requires moments when both partners simultaneously become vulnerable and open. Such risk-taking, though vitally important, cannot be accomplished if the couple experiences significant amounts of defensiveness and fear. Given their relationship history and legacy issues, the transition to intimacy would be quite difficult for them. Unable to move ahead on their own, they now need a setting that can sufficiently contain their anxieties to safely allow necessary levels of vulnerability and openness. Such an environment will allow them to look inward and gain insight into their intrapersonal issues and explore them in an open way. The current couples counseling situation is actually perceived and felt as threatening to both of them; it is feared that exposing elements of self would be used against them by their partner or would verify that they, alone, were the cause of the discord.

Severe Social and Vocational Issues

Because so much of our daily lives are consumed with work, job-related struggles often produce problems serious enough to disrupt other parts of our lives. In general, people find it exceedingly difficult to protect themselves and their families from work-related struggles. Western society places such a premium on success and productivity that many workers risk their health and their relationships as they respond to perceived and real work demands. A sluggish job market with increasing unemployment or underemployment levels only makes an already difficult situation, worse.

Stan works for his father-in-law. This working arrangement seemed ideal at the beginning of his career and relationship, but the years have brought increased conflict. Stan feels he could really improve the business but his recommendations "fall on deaf ears". His father-in-law has very narrow and definite ideas about how things need to be done so he refuses any of Stan's suggestions. Adding to his struggles, Stan recognizes similarities between his wife's and his father-in-law's personality when it comes to considering his recommendations. These personality characteristics frustrate him at work and at home. During his worst moments, he wonders how long he will be able to manage the reactions his father-in-law's stubbornness produces in him. He feels that he must suffer in silence since it is impossible for him to discuss his work-related concerns with his wife. The result is a collision between Stan's work and intimate relationships which leave him feeling paralyzed and minimized in both.

Lacy is grateful to her father for giving Stan a job and she knows that her husband would never have been able to land as good and as lucrative a position on his own. When she goes down this path of thinking, she also feels a lack of respect for Stan ("He would probably be unemployed if it weren't for my dad"). Equally devasting is the creeping thought that the job is just another example of how her dad is controlling her life. She remarks, "I can't really ask anything different from my relationship with my dad. If I upset him, he could fire Stan, and then she would be in real trouble. I feel paralyzed and responsible for the financial security of the family."

With both parties struggling with this issue and feeling helpless to do anything about it, they end up turning the issue towards the relationship. Neither one feels empowered to work the issues about with the correct person (boss or father), but they do feel capable of blaming each other for the conflict. The resulting impact is growing resentment and distance.

Unreasonable or Rigid Expectations of Counseling

Unreasonable or rigid expectations of counseling often result when a couple sheds individual and collective responsibility for their plight. They tend to expect the counselor, or the counseling process, to assume responsibility for change rather than themselves. Rigidity also indicates that the couple fears accepting responsibility for patterns or attitudes that may be distressing and blocking the couple from achieving desired levels of intimacy. Virtually, all high conflict couples enter counseling with unreasonable and rigid expectations. Some expect the counselor to determine who is right and wrong; others have concluded that their partner is the cause of the trouble and the one who needs to change. Such couples adhere to these beliefs with varying levels of intensity. As the intake process unfolds, their level of rigidity can and should be assessed because the clinician can use this level to estimate the amount and source of the couple's fears. These expectations challenge counselors in important ways. Inexperienced or unwitting counselors can respond to the client's fears by assuming more responsibility for the process than would be helpful, and they can align with one client or the other in very damaging ways.

This couple's prior counseling experiences offer a worrisome history. Each attempt failed to achieve the desired outcomes and left the couple more hopeless than when they began. Poor boundaries, coupled with a narrow clinical focus on the individuals rather than the relationship, contaminated both efforts. Of course, the couple's dynamics contributed to the problems, but the counselors share a much larger portion of the blame.

Unfortunately, Stan and Lacy now expect that only one of them will be satisfied with the counselor they choose. They expect to befriend any clinician they select and assume the therapy will somehow heal them without having to invest too much in the process. Instead of working together to find an appropriate counselor, they are desperately trying to find a referee, and they are more invested in finding a person who can verify their individual reality and prove "rightness" than they are in finding a relational pathway. This dynamic will often surface in session as the counselor attempts to build rapport with the clients. Consider the following interchange:

Dr. Levitov:	Lacy, you mentioned feeling unheard in the relationship. Tell me more about that.
Lacy:	No one listens to anything I say! It's like my opinion does not matter at all. I feel undermined all the time and don't feel taken seriously.
Dr. Levitov:	You would like to feel more respected in the relationship.
Lacy:	Yes! Thank you! That's the word: respect. <Stan is fidgeting in his chair and mumbles, "That's not true.">
Dr. Levitov:	I'm sorry Stan. I didn't hear you.
Stan:	I said that what she is saying isn't true.

Dr. Levitov: You feel you respect her.

Stan: Well, yeah, but I don't feel respected either. And it's like she's trying to paint this picture like I am the bad guy.

Dr. Levitov: When she expresses the need to be understood, you feel like you are being blamed for its absence?

Stan: Well, yeah. That's what she is saying, and no one is listening to me.

Dr. Levitov: So, there are times that you feel unheard and disrespected as well.

Stan: Exactly.

Lacy: Why are you listening to him? See, it always comes back to how *he* feels. What about me?

This example illustrates the common high conflict couple dynamic of intolerance for empathy shown to the partner. As the counselor utilizes rapport building skills needed in the early phases of counseling, the individual not in focus feels abandoned and unheard. It is as if empathy shown toward one member meant "taking sides". Counselors will feel this tug-of-war in session, and most will report how frustrating it is. As mentioned in Chapter 2, this dynamic is not unique to high conflict couples, but the intensity is. When encountered in most couples, the lack of tolerance of empathy toward the other partner can be handled by discussing the issue with the couple via a well-timed process observation. In these cases, the couple will accept the insight gained and be open to the counselor connecting with both of them to improve the relationship. In high conflict couples, the lack of tolerance will persist and the counselor will often experience some of the relationship patterns that are contributing to the disconnection. Here is one account from a supervisee who experienced this dynamic in counseling:

It was like there was only a certain amount of empathy I could give. As I poured the "cup" of empathy into one of them, the other experienced it as taking the empathy from their cup (stealing it) and giving it to the other. Then it happened again as I made an attending remark to the offended party. I kept thinking, "Empathy is not a finite resource. There is plenty to go around," but any empathy shared was perceived as betrayal.

Let's return to Stan and Lacy to see what this escalation might look like:

Dr. Levitov:	So, there are times that you feel unheard and disrespected as well.
Stan:	Exactly.
Lacy:	Why are you listening to him? See, it always comes back to how *he* feels. What about me?
Dr. Levtiov:	I'm noticing that it causes you some discomfort when I talk and validate Stan. And Stan, I noticed you start to get agitated when I try to understand Stacy.
Stan:	I didn't really notice.
Lacy:	Oh, this is complete bullshit. Are you kidding me? You are going to try some therapist sugar words to try to make us feel like we are doing something wrong? And of course, I am the bad one, right?
Dr. Levitov:	It's not a matter of who is to blame. It is important for all of us to understand the ways we are connecting and disconnecting from each other in our work. For us to make progress, I am going to need to be able to listen to each one of you and the other will not only need to learn to be okay with that focus of attention, but also learn to listen to each other as well.
Stan:	Hmmm. I guess so. I think we listen great.
Lacy:	See?! Stan isn't listening to a word you say. He's just agreeing to shut you up. And I know what you are saying. I don't listen and if I did better, everything would be fixed. It's bullshit. I can't take this. It's too much. I'm taking a break. (Lacy walks out).
Stan (to counselor):	I think you are doing a great job and we'll be fine.

Notice in this example how the intolerance escalates as the counselor continues the rapport building? The result is that it makes traditional couple's counseling much more difficult. In fact, as we have mentioned, these are the kinds of couples who either leave counseling, as they have done several times before or are referred and terminated under the "they aren't ready to change" rationale. We understand that all approaches of counseling would have a method for dealing with this and would conceptualize it in several ways. While those approaches are viable, we believe TCC has some advantages, which will be explained later.

In the end, empty promises made by previous counselors misled them; therapy can only offer a setting where they can try to improve their relationship and learn to help one another heal. Their counterproductive expectations, born of flawed previous attempts, jeopardize future efforts unless the new process (1) immediately and directly confronts their false assumptions and (2) replaces the previous unhealthy clinical relationships with well-bounded, professional, and effective interventions.

Step Three: The Transition to Individual Sessions

Once the decision to implement TCC is made, the couple must work with the current counselor to find a collaborating counselor to begin the individual sessions. In practices that routinely make TCC a part of their options, a group of prospects might be available which the clients can choose from. If you are just starting out, you might only have one or two mental health professionals that meet your own personal and professional guidelines for co-therapy, as outlined in Chapter 4. Regardless of your situation, you want to explain the rationale of the referral list and clearly identify the importance of the co-therapy relationship as part of the client's process of potential change.

Unless very compelling reasons to do otherwise, we let the couple select their counselors from the referral list provided. To accomplish this, we ask the couple to visit with the other counselor. They attend a fifty-minute intake session with the member of the team they have not yet met—they offer information about their relationship and direct their own questions to the counselor. In cases where one of the prospective counselors possesses expertise particularly well-suited to one of the clients, the suggestion to work with that client is made. Of course, the final decision rests with the couple but most of the time clients agree with the recommendation and follow it.

Assuming there are no reasons to suggest how the couple should be assigned, we simply give them the liberty to choose and contact the counselor they have selected. We rarely predict which counselor the clients will select. While we seldom understand the logic they use, their choices always seem to be insightful and quite correct—even in cases where choices initially seem mismatched, the wisdom of their selection surfaces within a short period of time. Oddly enough, it seems that even couples who are heavily conflicted can make particularly good choices about who to select as their counselor.

Step Four: Individual Sessions

Clients remain in individual therapy between four to eight weeks. This is not a fixed rule since some couples move very rapidly to joint sessions and others need more time. The final decision on when to begin the joint sessions usually rests on the counselors and comes from their consultations where each of the client's progress is evaluated. Prior to moving into joint sessions, each counselor must believe progress has been made in the following areas:

1 Rapport has been developed between counselor and client;
2 Counselor and client have insight into how intrapersonal issues have contributed to the relationship dynamics (both constructive and destructive); and
3 The client is skilled at focusing on self and has identified at least one personal change he/she can bring to the relationship dynamic.

An interesting irony developed over the years as we implemented the model: the couple's readiness for joint counseling turned out to be inversely proportional to their perceived and shared need to begin these sessions. In other words, whenever one of the couples start pestering their counselor to meet jointly, we discovered that they were not yet ready to do so. Since the need to manage anxiety in the joint sessions is so important, we must be sure that they would interact in effective ways.

When desperation to meet exists in either of the couple, we noticed that the neediness consistently propelled the joint process away from the desired outcomes. While critics may raise the concern that the couple is being deliberately delayed from obtaining relief from relationship problems, we have found that this is not the case. Most couples use their individually gained insights to explain themselves to their partners and they ask each other many questions about what they've learned in individual therapy. We rely upon the individual therapy gains to ensure that the couple's work will be as efficient and effective as possible. Starting before the couples are fully ready reduces joint session efficacy.

Each of the couple receives updates on their individual work along with a projected joint session schedule. They usually understand how the individual work translates into their relationship and they seem content by being able to work out individual concerns that had profound negative impact on their relationship. The relative safety of the individual session gives clients a chance to explore issues they previously greeted with defensiveness. Imagine how difficult it would be for Lacy to discuss her need for control, and the relationship of these patterns to those of her father, in front of Stan. Such control issues affect relationships, and the couple must, at some point, discuss them. However, counselors should prepare the couple so they can productively manage such important, emotionally charged topics.

Role of Co-therapy During the Individual Counseling Stage

TCC relies upon the ability of the counselors to relate to one another in an open and productive way. As we mentioned earlier, the relationship between the counselors is used to relate to the couple's relationship. To ensure that the process honors this concern from the outset, couples review and sign releases allowing the counselors to discuss information obtained in the individual sessions. The information discussed focuses on two crucial elements: (1) how the intrapersonal impacts the interpersonal and (2) how the information learned about the other client impacts the counselor. If I am Stan's counselor, I would be listening to information about Stacy through the lens of Stan. As I listen, I am paying attention to my thoughts and feelings about what I am hearing. These insights give me deeper information about Stan. I can then share those with my co-counselor and vice-versa. This process is vital and is unique to TCC.

The idea that dynamics from one relationship carries over inconsistent relational patterns into another relationship is referred to as a parallel process. Most often discussed in clinical supervision literature, it has a place in TCC. The parallel process concerns surface early in the TCC process. Themes and artifacts of the clients' conflicts infiltrate the counselors and their relationship as they consult with one another. We learned to fully appreciate the value of these disturbances in our consultative relationship because they completely illuminate the struggles the clients experience. For example, during consultation meetings Stan's counselor, echoing his client's patterns, tended to minimize concerns as Lacy's counselor pressed for control and the need for change in Stan's behavior. When counselors expect parallel process effects to surface, they work through the biases brought by the influence of their respective clients and craft an approach that honors their client's struggles more accurately. The journey can be perilous if counselors ignore the parallel process effects. Unhealthy triangulations where the counselor and client unite against the other pair severely inhibit the process. On the other hand, when these patterns are discussed rather than "acted out," clients obtain valuable insights about their relationship and they identify points where strengthening is possible. Paying attention and utilizing a parallel process is so important to TC, and we will discuss it further while providing examples throughout the next steps.

Stan and Lacy in Individual Sessions

Individual counseling can proceed by utilizing the counselor's preferred approach and orientation. The rapport building process for TCC is important and much easier to achieve in an individual session as compared to a couple's format. The counselor can fully focus on the individual without being undermined or distracted by some of the issues that occur in high conflict couples that make that process challenging, if not impossible. The focus here is two-fold:

1   Build a therapeutic alliance with each client based on healthy boundaries; and

2   Explore intrapersonal patterns and how changes to those patterns
     might produce interpersonal patterns.

To provide some sense of what might transpire in the individual sessions, we revisit Stan and Lacy and explore what their individual sessions focused on.

Stan

Stan had never been in individual counseling before and began by
mistrusting the process.

Dr. Fall:	Thanks for coming today, Stan. As we discussed, the purpose of these sessions is to focus on you and learn a bit about your patterns in your relationships.
Stan:	Yeah, as I said before, I don't know really what to say. I mean, I think Lacy is the one with the problem, or at least she's the one that thinks there is a problem.
Counselor:	So all of this must be confusing to you?
Stan:	Yes!
Counselor:	Maybe we can spend some time exploring the confusion and trying to get some clarity.
Stan:	I guess that sounds okay.

Here, the counselor is focusing on building rapport and connecting
the client with the process. Although the client tries to move the discussion to his wife, the counselor moves it back to his own feelings.
This sets the tone for the work as it moves forward. In the next four
sessions, the counselor explored Stan's family of origin issues and illuminated patterns that impacted Stan's relationship across his lifetime.
Pattern searching is useful because it helps the client see their role in the
interpersonal processes and prevents the client from thinking that the
circumstances are due to a sole "other". An individual session with Lacy
would have proceeded in the same way. To give you some clarity about
the desired outcome, summaries of both individuals are presented in
Tables 5.1 and 5.2.

Table 5.1 Stan's Individual Counseling Summary.

Key Relationships	Patterns of Connection/Disconnection
Father	Connect: via memories Disconnect: overwhelmed by loss; will deny the impact
Mother	Connect: not be a nuisance, be helpful, invisible Disconnect: same, withdraw, "Everything's fine"
Step-dads	Denied any relationship, "They are one big blob."
Father in Law	Connect: "Create no waves in the company." Disconnect: Avoid him
Lacy	Connect: "Try to make a stable home" "I make everything okay"
	Disconnect: feel hurt, stupid, and tends to shut down when feeling overwhelmed

Patterns identified:

Fear of negativity and negative consequences

Understands that terrible things happen (death of the father; mom's multiple failed relationships, etc.) but doesn't understand why they happen.

They developed strategies of ignoring issues to minimize or avoid the impact. The more someone illuminates a problem, the more he will deny. In past relationships, this pattern usually causes others to leave, which makes the "problem" go away. In his current relationship, Lacy is not going away (or hasn't yet) and he also cares about the relationship, so he feels stuck.

Points of possible personal change:

Gain insight into the pattern

Gain insight into the advantages and disadvantages of pattern

Identify modifications in approach:

- Openness to discuss issues; be proactive vs reactive
- Use relationship as support for dealing with problems vs seeing Lacy as an opponent
- Risk holding contact with "negative" feedback or events

To give some insight into how co-counselor collaboration is used, the following examples help illuminate that process.

Co-counselor Consult #1

This consult occurred after the second individual session. Keep in mind, each counselor is sharing information and is listening through the lens of their respective client and providing present perceptions to deepen the understanding about patterns in the couple's relationship.

Table 5.2 Lacy's Individual Counseling Summary.

Key Relationships	Patterns of Connection/Disconnection
Father	Connect: try to please Disconnect: feel controlled; argue, fight
Mother	Connect: be helpful; direct her Disconnect: criticism; judgmental, then guilt
Sister	Connect: share feelings, talk, vulnerability Disconnect: fight, yell
Stan	Connect: Try to support him; motivator Disconnect: feel ignored, so I yell at him, call him names, withhold affection.

Patterns identified:
Feels torn between not liking the feeling of being controlled but uses control to impact others.
See her role in relationships as being a "motivator".
Lacy seems scared of being perceived as "weak" like her mom, but also doesn't want to hurt others via control like her dad. When she feels weak, which occurs when she feels unheard, disrespected, not valued, she responds with criticism. As she becomes critical, she is aware she sounds like her father and gets angry and frustrated. This comes out as more intense criticism and controlling behavior, which often escalates into extreme feelings of being ignored or neglected.

Points of possible personal change:
Gain insight into the pattern
Gain insight into the advantages and disadvantages of pattern
Identify modifications in approach:

• Creating a space to listen to others
• Develop the skill of encouraging as a motivator which can be a connection-based motivator vs. criticism which is more disjunctive.
• Learn to modulate the intensity of criticism, anger, and guilt

Dr. Levitov: Okay, things are going well with Lacy. I find her incredibly open and willing to discuss her perspective.

Dr. Fall: Likewise with Stan. There was a bit of resistance with focusing on himself, but I think he is appreciating and liking the ability to talk about himself.

Dr. Levitov: Good. Sounds like the individual process is working! I think I'd like to share some things I have learned about Lacy and then we can go from there. Does that sound okay?

Dr. Fall: Sure. I will try to listen as Stan and see what comes up.

Dr. Levitov: Great. Lacy has explored her relationship in her family of origin. She sees herself as torn between loving her parents and loathing them. She admires her mom's dedication to family but also sees her as spineless and without a "real" identity. She admires her father's work ethic and strong identity but also sees him as demanding and stifling. She is sure she takes elements from both but feels stuck in the middle. She feels insecure and that often comes out in criticism and control.

Dr. Fall: Okay. Yeah, I think Stan would sense that in the relationship, and he would be sensitive to the criticism and take it personally. I don't think he would empathize with it. As I am listening, it was the last sentence that really stuck out to me and I think it's because I started thinking about myself (as Stan) and just blew all the other stuff that didn't directly impact me. In our sessions, Stan explored his family, but he really strives to make everything okay, steering away from pain. For example, his father's death and his mom's multiple marriages were summed up with, "I was too young to really know what was going on." It's like that part of his life is locked away in a box. He tends to try to put a positive spin on everything.

Dr. Levitov: That's really frustrating.

Dr. Fall: You are feeling frustrated?

Dr. Levitov: Yes. It's like he can't take anything seriously. He minimizes everything. I mean the suicide of his dad when he was 8? No impact?! Don't you think that seriously gets in his way of changing?

Dr. Fall: Sure. But he also contributes a lot to the family. He's not all bad (laughs).

Dr. Levitov: Right. I didn't say he was all bad. Let's talk about what is happening here.

Dr. Fall: Good idea. Tell me about your feelings of frustration.

Dr. Levitov: I think I felt like there was an opportunity for him. That if he could just acknowledge what's going on around him, then he could change. I think Lacy perceives that "positive spin" as minimizing and she doesn't feel understood. She then gets frustrated and uses criticism or directives to jar him loose.

Dr. Fall: Interesting. As you got more frustrated, I felt the need to be more positive, so maybe that's an aspect of balance that is occurring in the relationship. They are both trying to balance each other, but it's just perpetuating the cycle.

Dr. Levitov: That's useful information to use in our work.

Co-counselor Consult #2

This consult occurred after the fourth session.

Dr. Levitov: Okay, things are progressing nicely on this front. Lacy is doing a wonderful job focusing on herself and is getting close to being able to talk about change without switching over to what Stan can do differently. How about you?

Dr. Fall: I might need a little more time. I think two more sessions would be beneficial and he agrees. He has opened up about his father's death and I think he is making some connections between that and his relationship with his father-in-law and those insights are beginning to attach to his relationship with Lacy.

Dr. Levitov: Sounds good. Lacy is gaining a greater understanding of her use of criticism in her relationships. She seems to try to use it as a motivator for others. She feels strong when she does it even when she knows it hurts someone.

Dr. Fall: If someone isn't motivated by the criticism, what does she do?

Dr. Levitov: What most people do... she criticizes more.

Dr. Fall: As she does that, I want to just keep moving away. In some ways, I also want to talk about all the things that are going well.

Dr. Levitov: Right. I would perceive that as avoidance and minimization, which might lead to criticizing you more. It's weird, but when you were talking about needing more time individually, my first instinct was to try to make you go faster... by criticizing you. Now that thought makes more sense.

Dr. Fall: I think Stan is beginning to see that the positive spin technique has some advantages, but that it also costs him and his relationships. Sometimes when I hear you talk, especially when you are critical, I can actually feel the fear of everything falling apart. I wonder if that's part of what his dynamic is about. If he doesn't inject positivity, his entire world will come crashing down—Lacy will leave, he will lose his job, and his kids will hate him.

Dr. Levitov: Okay, we can keep working on this and start talking about meeting as a couple in a few weeks.

Both examples demonstrate the appropriate and effective use of co-counselor consults. The information helps facilitate movement toward the couple's work and the use of parallel process deepens the insight of both intrapersonal and interpersonal dynamics that can impact the clients. While these were examples of how a parallel process can be used effectively, not being aware of this dynamic allows the toxic elements of the couple's relationship to come crashing into the co-counselor relationship. The last example demonstrates what inattention to parallel process might look like.

Co-counselor Consult: Ignorance of Parallel Process

Dr. Levitov: Okay, things are progressing nicely on this front. Lacy is doing a wonderful job focusing on herself and is getting close to being able to talk about change without switching over to what Stan can do differently. How about you?

Dr. Fall: I might need a little more time. I think two more sessions would be beneficial and he agrees. He has

opened up about his father's death and I think he
is making some connections between that and his
relationship with his father-in-law and those insights
are beginning to attach to his relationship with Lacy.

Dr. Levitov: Well, I sort of feel like he should be ready. Lacy has
been working really hard and I don't think she is going
to want to wait around for another month. Should I just
terminate with her for a month and you can let us know
when he's ready?

Dr. Fall: Hmmm.... well I'm not sure if her being out of
counseling for a month would be good. Maybe there's
other work to be done? I don't know. He is working
hard and making progress too. Just last week he really
dove into the material with his dad. It was exciting.

Dr. Levitov: That's great and all, but that's sort of his pattern, right?
He'll be telling her everything is going well and "work is
being done," but meanwhile, nothing is really changing
at home and she's left to wait for him to get his shit
together.

Dr. Fall: I know the timeline is not in sync, but the sky isn't
falling either: he's working, she's working. Just at
different speeds. Maybe if she was less focused on
his work and more on her own, this might go better.
Also, it's not a race. She needs to chill.

Dr. Levitov: It's hard to chill when your marriage is falling apart, and
your husband seems content to slowly explore issues
that should have been dealt with years ago.

Hopefully, the differences in this co-counselor consult are apparent. In
this example, the co-counselors are not paying attention to the parallel
process dynamics and as a result, are acting out the client dynamics
within the co-counselor relationship. The lack of awareness will likely
result in a deteriorating co-counselor relationship which may lead to
negative consequences in the client's work, especially if the work
progressed into joint sessions. Awareness of the parallel process allows
the counselors to make use of that dynamic and gain a richer perspective
on the client's issue, which can then be relayed back to the clients.

It is important to note that although we gave you a couple of examples here, consultations typically occur frequently, often on a weekly basis, during both the individual and later tandem sessions. As mentioned in Chapter 4, consistent interaction between the co-therapists is a hallmark of quality co-therapy. The consultations provide a way to monitor the progress of the couple as well as make full use of the co-therapy relationship in that process. Lastly, it provides the time needed to work on and nurture the co-therapy relationship. If you are doing co-therapy and not meeting with your partner on a regular basis, you are missing the full potential of the modality and at worst, you could be doing damage to your clients.

Step Five: Couples Are Readied for the Joint Sessions

The preliminary individual sessions help clients identify the personal issues that may be adversely affecting their relationship, support them as they unearth concerns, develop plans for change, and identify resources that will be helpful to their personal efforts and their relationship. This explicit relationship focus differentiates TCC preliminary individual counseling from individual counseling in general. Within the relative safety individual sessions afford, clients gain insights about how their family-of-origin experiences affect their partner. They begin to realize how easily they misunderstand or misinterpret one another and how much energy it takes to correct their assumptions. We confirm these changes by directly observing the client as he or she correctly surmises the impact their legacies have on their relationship, and when they tell us about the discussions they initiate with their partner. In individual sessions, clients not only realize how each partner's legacy issues affect the relationship but they begin to see how intertwined the patterns have become.

We often use the term "corners" to illustrate an antagonistic intertwining of relationship issues. Virtually, all couple relationships rely on these corners to manage anxiety internally or externally, affecting the relationship. In Stan and Lacy's case, the corners were labeled by each person as:

Stan: Positive Land

Lacy: Criticism

Each party will be sensitive to the manifestations of the other person's strategy which results in choosing their own corner behavior. So, when Stan perceives Criticism, he moves to Positive Land, which leads Lacy to plow further deeper into criticism. If Lacy chooses Criticism, Stan will promptly move to Positive Land. It's important to note that each one feels the other is to blame. Stan will say, "If Lacy wasn't so critical, I wouldn't have to focus so much on the positive" and Lacy will say, "If Stan could take things seriously, I wouldn't have to point out what needs to be done so much." Both may be right, from a behavioral cycle perspective, but the problem is that neither understands the personal responsibility they have for impacting their individual choices. The cycle is further complicated as each of the couple relied on each other's own interpretations— ones that are based on their family of origin. The history, as it combines with the emotionality already present in the relationship, makes it very difficult for partners to see one another clearly. Seeing these patterns, understanding the patterns, and being accountable for how each can change the pattern are the necessary elements for moving into the joint sessions.

As might be evident, planning for the joint sessions begins as soon as the individual sessions start. Each counselor develops hypotheses about their client and the clients' relationship. Consultations invite the counselors to discuss their findings and refine their assumptions about the couple, the couple's struggles, and their resources. Because individual sessions produce a wealth of important information about each partner, counselors quickly identify the couple's relationship themes and patterns of interaction. Armed with this information, counselors better anticipate where conflicts arise, how partners tend to misunderstand each other, the effects of each partner's history on the relationship, and possible directions to pursue if intimacy is to successfully replace conflict.

As the counselors begin to sense that the individuals are ready to meet jointly, this shift is discussed with each client. It is common for this discussion to produce some anxiety in the clients. Fear of "being ready" and moving out of the comfort of the individual sessions and into the unknown of the couple's sessions are typical topics for exploration. Keep in mind that each client is holding a perception of couple's counseling based on past experiences rife with failure and conflict, so it is normal for them to be apprehensive. The advantage of TCC is that each client brings with them a counselor who understands them at a deep level. Reflecting on the work accomplished in the individual sessions can provide support and hope for the couple's sessions. It is also important to note that the approach to the couple's sessions will be different from previous experiences. Namely, each client is coming in and will express what they have learned about themselves and how those patterns impact the relationship. Even more importantly, each person will identify what they can change to produce a different outcome. This is vastly different from the typical, "I am in pain; this is what you can do differently" dynamic that gets played out in other forms of couple's therapy.

Step Six: Tandem Sessions

As the couple begins their work in tandem sessions, we outline the basic goals and rules to avoid any confusion and help the couple settle into the pattern that will form the remainder of their therapy. We remind them that all our efforts will be focused on helping understand their relationship and implementing better ways of becoming responsible stewards of the relationship. We stress that a healthy relationship is probably the best gift they could give one another—and the most important gift that they could offer to their children. We remind them that in the tandem sessions there are no restrictions on patterns of interaction—counselors and clients are free to speak to and offer questions to anyone they choose. While the individual sessions were conducted with one counselor and one client, the tandem sessions open the range of possible interactions within what has now become a small group. The results are quite interesting and revealing. For example, some clients will pose questions to their partner's therapist that unearth interesting concerns that are unlikely to surface in conventional couples counseling (or ones that surface only after a protracted period of time). One client asked her partner's counselor how he perceived her based on his interaction with her husband. Her question allowed her to assess how her husband thought about her and how those thoughts might impact the counselor's view of her. This mode of getting information about someone else's perspective by speaking to a third party eventually became a focus of our work in the tandem therapy. The woman was raised in a family where her father was inaccessible, so she and all of her siblings learned about dad through interactions with mom. For obvious reasons, this kind of proxy relationship created many problems in their couple relationship.

Stress a Focus on the Relationship

Almost immediately, we introduce the idea that all behavior should be consistently evaluated in terms of how it affects the relationship. For any considered behavior, we suggest a simple test: Did the actions improve, have no impact on, or hurt the relationship? While the test is simple on the surface, its usefulness is remarkable as it can be applied to any situation. We found it helpful to begin this process of considering how individual choices impact the relationship during the individual sessions, once the client is comfortable with focusing on themselves, providing a nice bridge into the joint sessions and prevents self-centeredness. One technique we use is to ask the clients to consider the couple as a third entity, like a pet or even their yard. We know it sounds funny, but here is how the discussion might go:

> Counselor: You have done really good work identifying how your pattern of responding to anxiety in the relationship leads you to choose behaviors of isolation.
>
> Client: Yeah. I can definitely see how that behavior protects me but also cuts me off from the attention I really want to happen. I want my partner to show she loves me by coming and finding me and dragging me out of my hole. When that doesn't happen, I feel rejected.
>
> Counselor: Great points. With this insight, we can begin to think about how those choices impact not only you but your partner and the relationship.
>
> Client: Cool.
>
> Counselor: I want you to consider thinking about your relationship as a third entity in your life. Some clients like to think of

	it as a pet, a child, or even their lawn. It's something that exists outside of you and your partner, but both of you will have responsibilities tending and nurturing it.
Client:	Oh, it's got to be our cat. We both love Ruby! That would be easy for us to think about.
Counselor:	Ok. We decide on the joint target later, but for now, it sounds like Ruby the cat works for you.
Client:	Yes.
Counselor:	Now, every time we are exploring an event in your life and the possible choices, we view it in three different ways: what you need, what your partner needs, and what the relationship needs. We can also hypothesize about the impact of the choices and explore mutual goals. Does that make sense?
Client:	Sure. So, like, if I want to go play soccer at a tournament for the weekend — I want to go and have fun — my partner might have other plans. She wants to have fun too. Or she might have to work; she needs to work and make money.
Counselor:	What about Ruby?
Client:	Well, we have to make sure she is taken care of.
Counselor:	How do you do that?
Client:	By talking and planning.
Counselor:	Exactly. Would there ever be a situation where you both decide that having fun and making money are more important than Ruby? The result being she is going to starve this weekend.
Client:	Oh, no way! We would figure it out.
Counselor:	Right, you would figure out a way to take care of her and probably still get a little fun and work. So, that's how I want you to start considering the relationship.
Client:	Wow... I don't think I do that now. When relationship needs come up, I feel like I have to give something up to tend to the relationship and I fight it.

This paradigm allows them to consider and balance the needs of self, others, and the relationship and makes it much easier to identify and work toward a mutual goal. Of course, there are times when individual needs must take precedence, but they are nowhere near as frequent as we tend to believe they are. Unfortunately, many couples fear that their needs will not be met, and these individual needs create something of a continuous competition within the couple to either of their needs met. This type of conflict creates a place where the relationship will never be able to flourish.

In little time clients learn to start sessions with almost no prompting by offering comments like "I really helped the relationship earlier this week by remembering our anniversary and planning a surprise night out for my spouse" or "There were several things I could have done this week to help the relationship but chose not to, and while it didn't hurt the relationship I missed chances to improve it." There are the inevitable comments that usually begin with one partner saying to the other partner something like "Go ahead and tell the counselors what you did Friday night!" The partner then describes an evening where he or she drank to excess, used drugs, acted out sexually, or gambled. Once acknowledgment of offending behaviors is delivered, clients almost always answer the inevitable question often without prompting—they quickly admit that they hurt the relationship. This acceptance refocuses the couple on their goal of improving the relationship, and while it holds the offending partner responsible, it dramatically diminishes the potential for the non-productive shaming that often accompanies such behavior in most settings. We also avoid situations where we have to be the arbiters of what is good and bad because couples almost always make accurate judgments of a behavior's impact upon the relationship. The same cannot be said about an individual's evaluation of their own behavior mainly because defensiveness and fear are too intense. In simple terms, it is easier to say, "What I did hurt the relationship" than it is to say, "I am a bad person."

We also suggest that there may be times when clients may need to forgo one or more of what they perceive as their own needs in favor of caring more immediately for the needs of the relationship. High conflict couples often see this idea as a threat. In our society, personal needs often take precedence over communal needs as a result of established cultural patterns and advertising efforts. Once they experience the effects of intimacy that arise from caring for the relationship, they modify their perspective, though it often takes time as it requires a leap of faith.

One hard-working client who tended not to be as fond of dogs as his wife offered this story: He would come home late after a long day at work and his wife would suggest that they walk the dog. He would immediately sense the resistance to the idea of just sitting down and watching the news on the television. He stated to himself, "Walking a dog is the last thing I want to do, but my relationship needs a dog walk so I will." The dog walk allowed him and his wife to share their day, discuss their concerns, talk about their family, and develop much-needed plans for how they would spend time with one another. The relationship benefits were immediately reinforcing and he became more skilled in acting in favor of the relationship, as did his wife.

In Vivo Consultations

Tandem sessions offered us some unique opportunities to work with couples in ways that were previously impossible. In vivo consultation is one example that is unique to TCC. While there may be some models that utilize co-therapy from time to time, TCC is unique in its synthesis of best practices from literature on co-therapy and group co-leadership models, that focus on the co-therapy relationship as an agent of change. By purposefully using co-therapy this way, we could model cooperation toward a specific goal and let clients hear—and hopefully value—our professional discussion of their struggle.

The very first time we experimented with this option, we immediately realized its great potential. Confused about where we should proceed in the therapy, we looked toward each other and shared that we needed a few minutes to discuss the progress of the therapy. The couple granted us the permission we requested, and we began to discuss how things were going, what we should probably do next, and how we could support this new focus. The intensity of the couples' attention to our discussion defies description; they literally hung on each word. They listened carefully to how we linked each client's history to the current impasse. They nodded approval when we sympathized with each client's struggle to overcome their family of origin issues and toward the end, one client began to sob.

When we finished consulting after two or three minutes, we turned back to them for comments. They were clearly moved by the process. The tearful client said compassion filled her as she came to realize how much pain her husband had experienced in his early life. She recognized how difficulties early in his life were inhibiting his ability to relate, but he was trying. He was impressed with how the two counselors used their relationship to solve an important problem without fighting or having one stomp out of the room. This early reaction became commonplace over time, and the collection of these uniformly positive responses to in vivo consultations reinforced their continuous use. The process humanized the counselors as well—we were now more appropriately seen as people who did not have all the answers, yet are willing to struggle with what information we have as we sought to help our clients.

One final example bears mentioning at this point. One couple that endured a great deal of conflict in their relationship regularly posed challenging questions to each of us in the course of their TCC. We asked for a moment as we began an in vivo consultation. Ironically, as we discussed our concerns, we became defensive and somewhat annoyed with one another. The wife immediately picked up on the conflict and said, "Look at what we have done to their relationship." She had correctly identified the parallel process (mentioned earlier in the chapter) that was now inhabiting our clinical relationship. We stopped for a moment as she began to cry. We asked about the tears and her feelings of sadness. She readily admitted that the toxicity of their relationship had not only affected the counselors, but it was ever more seriously affecting and damaging their children. As we previously suggested, firsthand experiences on how a couple's relationship may affect others can be a very powerful change agent.

In providing training for TCC, the aspect of in vivo consultations seem to cause the most confusion and stress on counselors. The typical initial response is, "I would be comforted by having a colleague in session with me, but I have to talk to them?" Yes, you have to if you want to maximize the impact of co-therapy. Some examples with Stan and Lacy will help illustrate common uses of the in vivo consultation.

In Vivo Consultation #1

Stan:	I am feeling really vulnerable right now. I feel like I am sharing but I don't know if anyone is really hearing me, or if you think I'm crazy.
Dr. Fall:	So you feel you are stretching yourself, as we discussed, but you are wondering about how we are perceiving that.
Stan:	Yeah.
Lacy:	Well, I appreciate you being here and talking more. I do notice that.
Stan:	Okay. But do you think I'm being vulnerable and addressing negative things?
Lacy:	Yes ... and no. I mean, there are things we still need to work on—I don't want you to get the idea that we are done with this. There is still a long way to go. <starts fidgeting in her chair and wringing her hands>
Dr. Levtiov:	I would like to ask for a couple of minutes to talk with Dr. Fall. You can listen to what we say and then we will talk about it, okay?
Stan and Lacy:	Okay,
Dr. Levitov:	I am seeing something here that I want to check out with you.
Dr. Fall:	Okay/
Dr. Levitov:	I hear Stan asking for feedback on his level of sharing and risk. I see this as a change with him and is aligned with his goals. He is working hard on taking those risks and considering what he, Lacy, and the relationship needs.
Dr. Fall:	I agree. I hear Lacy wanting to affirm him, but there is also hesitation there. Almost as if she is afraid that if she says he is doing it, that he'll think everything is fine and stop.

Dr. Levitov:	Yes! And she's caught, because she wants to support him, but is worried the support won't be enough to motivate him to continue. I was worried if we didn't point this out, she might get anxious enough to revert to the old pattern of criticizing him.
Dr. Fall:	Interesting. I'm glad we talked about it. I'm also a little curious about the purpose of Stan's question. Internally, I had a brief sensation of wanting to applaud his efforts. When I felt that, my immediate thought was wondering if that was the purpose of his question: to get praise so he could feel like everything was okay. That's the old pattern.
Dr. Levitov:	Hmmm... I hadn't even thought of that. I want to hear their thoughts on our questions. Stan and Lacy, tell us what jumped out for you in this interchange.

In Vivo Consultation #2

Lacy:	I think things have really been improving lately. I have been calmer and at peace. I think Stan is doing a great job addressing things before I can even think of them, in some cases.
Dr. Levitov:	That sounds like progress. What have you been doing to contribute to this change?
Lacy:	I have tried to focus on positive interactions with the kids, my father, and Stan. I do think about the relationship more now—and not always in terms of what is wrong—about what is right and how I can make progress, if that makes sense.
Stan:	That's good to hear.
Lacy:	I do wonder if we could be doing more, or if this is it?
Dr. Levitov:	You are wondering where to go from here? Lacy: Right. I mean, this is great, but I have to think there is more to do.

Dr. Fall:	Stan, what are you feeling when you hear Lacy's perspective?
Stan:	I don't know. <fidgets>. I mean, I think she's saying everything else great?
Dr. Fall:	I would like to consult with Dr. Levitov for a moment.
Lacy and Stan:	Okay.
Dr. Fall:	I'm a little torn here so I wanted to process a bit. On one hand, I am happy that Lacy sees progress. On the other, I feel this pressure in my gut when she quickly moves to think about what else needs to change; I feel restless and conflicted. Like, can't we just be satisfied with the progress for a while?
Dr. Levitov:	I see what you're saying. It's difficult for you to tease out whether she is merely asking *if* there is anywhere else to go, or quickly becoming dissatisfied with the progress and wanting more.
Dr. Fall:	Yes, I think that's it.
Dr. Levitov:	I think you are in tune with Stan's perspective and considering his response, he seems to be feeling some discomfort and moving back to his Positive Land corner. Maybe it would be good for you to check out your perspective with Lacy, and Stan could benefit from watching how these issues could be processed.
Dr. Fall:	Great idea.

In both examples, the counselors are using their knowledge of the couple's dynamics to illuminate them in the present. This process is even more potent as it bypasses the couple's natural defense because of the alliance formed through the individual session processing. Instead of hearing the feedback and immediately increasing the intensity of defense, the clients feel more deeply seen and understood. Even when clients see the process differently, it can openly be discussed as the focus is not on correctness but understanding.

Early experiences with the use of in vivo consultation also illustrated an abstract and important reality. In this form of counseling, the relationship between the couple would often interact with the relationship between the counselors. While the couples lack a language to describe the phenomenon, they clearly experienced it and seemed usually comforted by it. We came to understand that this new paradigm contained more anxiety than traditional couples counseling and allowed the couples to take more risks as they explored the intimacy we targeted from the outset.

Role-playing by the Counselors

Having two counselors in the therapy room also permitted us to explore the use of role-playing exercises. Role-playing is similar to in vivo consultation — both utilize the co-therapy relationship to explore client dynamics. However, they differ in focus. Role-playing is typically a targeted approach focused on illuminating a specific dynamic or skill, while in vivo uses the co-therapy relationship to highlight couple patterns. Each of us had exhaustively interviewed our assigned clients in the early individual sessions as a prelude to the Tandem Counseling Sessions. We knew their patterns, history, and now could see their modes of interacting. Armed with such information, role-playing was a natural next step as long as (1) we selected useful scenarios to portray, (2) the clients agreed to the process, and (3) they would likely benefit from the activity.

Early experiences with role-playing also produced very positive results. Watching someone else portray their conflict from the other side of the room gave deep insights into how they appeared to us and one another. Here again, couples quickly identified with the counselors playing as actors, and they easily extrapolated what they saw to how their friends and family must feel when exposed to such conflict from them. They could also more easily pick out the family of origin patterns that haunted their relationship. Clients might say, "When you portray me, I can so easily see how I am acting like my father and how difficult that must be for my partner," or they might quip, "Your version of me was perfect and now I can even see ways to improve as I see where the problems may be." Of course, role-playing is not new to counseling but using it in such a controlled setting to help couples is a unique application.

On rare occasions, couples would actually ask us to act out elements of their relationship. They had so much trouble seeing what we were seeing; the graphic presentation proved intensely valuable. One couple introduced us to even more direct use of role-play. This couple asked us to act out their conflict first and then demonstrate how a couple that was able to properly cooperate would handle the problem. They perceived the obvious value of linking modeling and role-play activities in a way we had unfortunately overlooked. Role-playing examples with Stan and Lacy are included below.

Role-playing Example #1

Lacy:	I'm not sure what you mean by "corners". I think I get the idea that we both choose certain behaviors when we get upset, but I don't get how those are related. I think I get so focused on what he's doing that I lose the bigger picture.
Dr. Fall:	Yes, that is the function of corner behavior. Would it be helpful for Dr. Levitov and I to act out that dynamic for you?
Lacy:	Yes, that would be interesting. Dr. Levitov gets to play me? (laughs)
Dr. Levitov:	Yes, I will do my best and you can help modify if I get anything wrong. Stan, you can be Dr. Fall's coach.
Dr. Fall:	Okay, here we go (turns to Dr. Levitov). Hi Lacy, how is your day going?
Dr. Levitov:	It's okay; I have a lot on my plate today. I could use your help if you are not busy.
Dr. Fall:	Hmmm... I was hoping to relax today. I have been pretty busy at work this week.
Dr. Levitov:	Relax? We have that tax issue to take care of. We can't keep putting it off.
Dr. Fall:	Oh, that's no big deal. I'll get Bob to take a look at it.
Dr. Levitov:	Bob already looked at it and gave us the stuff to do. You can't keep putting everything off on other people.

	I'm getting sick of your shit, Stan. You are lazy and I can't keep picking up all the slack.
Dr. Fall:	Hmmm... sorry? I got a text and was reading it. We got invited to a party tonight, wanna go?
Dr. Levitov:	You are such a piece of shit, Stan.
Dr. Fall:	Why are you always so pissed off? I just asked you to go to a party and have fun, and you freak out.
Dr. Levitov:	This might be a good time to stop. What did you notice in the interchange?
Lacy:	Yes, that was great. I noticed that it escalated. Both of you became more intense in your approach.
Stan:	Yeah, I could see Lacy getting more and more agitated and me just fading out.
Dr. Fall:	You were aware of the connection between the two dynamics. As Lacy becomes more critical, you become more tuned out; as you become more tuned out, Lacy becomes more critical.
Lacy:	I see it now. We do that all the time. That's accurate.
Dr. Fall:	Would either of you modify anything in the role play? How would it be more accurate?
Lacy:	I am typically screaming at some point. You weren't mean enough (laughs).
Stan:	I normally walkout. That's my ultimate form of disappearing.

This example is a standard role play in TCC. It is often useful for couples to see their patterns in action early on in the joint sessions. The individual sessions produce the initial insight and the role-play tends to bring that insight to another level. Once the couple truly understands the interrelated nature of their choices, the exploration of alternatives becomes a natural pivot point. It is also important to note the importance of giving the couple an opportunity to modify and revise the role-play. This collaboration creates an active engagement of the role-playing process, rather than a passive "we are watching a movie" perspective. In the next example, we take the collaboration process a step further by having the clients act as real-time consultants to the role play. The couple is encouraged to actively give feedback to the role players and may even take a moment to have an in vivo consultation with each other or either counselor.

Role-playing Example #2

Stan:	I think I keep getting stuck with what I am supposed to be doing differently. I can clearly see what I want to do—the old pattern—but when I take that away, nothing else is really there. The result is just standing there, paralyzed, and I think that comes across as me doing nothing—which is the old pattern!
Dr. Fall:	You would like some help with generating alternatives and creating a new pattern.
Stan:	Yes.
Dr. Levitov:	Okay, we can role-play that scenario. As we do that, you will provide suggestions on what to do, how you're feeling as we choose certain behaviors or responses, and feel free to talk to each other if you need to.
Dr. Fall:	Okay, let's begin (turns to Dr. Levitov). Hey Lacy, can we talk about the credit card bill that's due on Monday?
Dr. Levitov:	You haven't paid for it yet?
Stan:	Okay, this is what I'm talking about. Dr. Fall, I would normally feel attacked by that, but it's just a question—and a simple one, really.
Dr. Fall:	You are aware of feeling attacked, but instead of moving forward with feeling attacked, you want to perceive it in a different way. If you perceived it as Lacy needing clarification, what would you do?
Stan:	I guess I would answer the question and stay focused on paying the bill.
Dr. Fall:	Nice. You have identified paying the bill as a possible

	mutual goal. Let's continue in that direction (turns back to Dr. Levitov). No, I haven't. I wanted to check in with you before I paid it to make sure we are on the same page.
Dr. Levitov:	Okay, that makes sense. What did you want to talk about?
Dr. Fall:	There are some charges here from Starbucks ... about $100 worth. I thought we agreed to cut back on that.
Stan:	Can I consult with Lacy for a moment?
Dr. Levitov:	Sure!
Stan:	That last comment made me really anxious; I don't think I could ever say that to you.
Lacy:	It's funny you say that. I felt my urge to attack you rising in my guts (laughs). But, if we agree on something and I am not doing it, I want you to feel that you can talk to me about it. Bringing it up would be a change for you; it's your job to take the risk and it's mine not to attack you for doing it, I think.
Stan:	That makes sense. Can you guys role play that to show us what it might look like?
Dr. Fall:	Sure. I'll restate the last part. There are some charges here from Starbucks... about $100 worth. I thought we agreed to cut back on that.
Dr. Levitov:	When I hear that, I want to argue with you, but I'm going to try to listen instead.
Dr. Fall:	Okay, good. I'm glad (laughs). I mean, I'm not trying to attack you either. I'm just pointing out something that we agreed on and see if anything has changed.
Dr. Levitov:	No, you are right. I just lost track of what I was doing. I think I was feeling like a deserved a treat and so I went to Starbucks.
Dr. Fall:	I agree you deserve treats. The purpose of our plan wasn't to deny ourselves stuff but to be more disciplined about money.

Dr. Levitov: Thanks for not making me feel bad about it.

Lacy: Okay, that sounds good and actually feels good too. However, at the end of the day, I violated the agreement and nothing has really changed.

Dr. Levitov: You are thinking you should be punished?

Lacy: Hmmm, I guess so.

Dr. Fall: The role of the relationship is not to punish, but to connect with one another when things are going well and when things get shaky. The idea here is that you will work together to stay focused on the things you feel are best for the relationship and work together to correct behaviors that aren't healthy for the relationship.

Stan: I see what you're saying. I can't stop her from spending money and I don't want to be in that position anyway. Instead, we use the relationship to motivate us.

Dr. Levitov: That's a great point.

Overall, role-plays provide an excellent method for working with the complicated dynamics of a high conflict couple within a TCC format. The knowledge gained and rapport built in the individual sessions create a safe atmosphere to quickly and effectively work with the couple from a number of interesting perspectives. Co-counselors who are using their relationship properly will feel comfortable interacting with each other freely, and the couple will gain deeper levels of insight by seeing the dynamic in action and playing an active role in participating in the role plays.

Information Sharing

In all forms of counseling, it is common to find skills deficits that inhibit the desired progress toward the client's goals. In these situations, it is appropriate to impart information that might be helpful to the client. The information chosen should be offered in a collaborative manner and should be connected to the struggles and goals of the client. Some common concepts that often come up in TCC include:

1   Information about concepts found in General Systems Theory such as triangulation, individuation, boundary dynamics, hierarchies, and homeostasis. We have found that these elements provide a useful context for couples within the TCC approach and most can be conceptualized with other existing theoretical frameworks.

2   Information about the different types of intimacy can be helpful in expanding the couple's perspective on building intimacy. For example, exploring how to create spiritual, intellectual, and emotional intimacy and compatibility in the relationship helps broaden the couple's options for deepening the relationship in ways that were previously unknown to the couple. (Fall & Howard, 2017). Clients have told us that they enjoy *The Dance of Intimacy* (Lerner, 1997) as a resource that helped them understand gender issues in intimacy.

3   Information about parenting can be helpful when the couple is also participating in the parent role. Patterns that surface within the couple will also be expressed in the parent-child relationship. Learning about healthy parenting strategies can be woven into the change process and have a positive impact on multiple levels within the family. Some common resources include *Positive Discipline A-Z* (Nelson, 2006); *No-Drama Discipline* (Siegel & Bryson, 2016); and *How to Talk so your Kids will Listen and Listen so Kids will Talk* (Faber & Mazlish, 2012).

4   Information about sexuality can be useful to the couple, as conflict within the relationship can be expressed within their sexual relationship. We also know that problems associated with sexuality can then manifest in other facets of the relationship. Openly talking about sexuality is important for couples and should be modeled within the counseling relationship. Resources needed here can vary from information about health-related issues, communicating about sexuality within the relationship, and improving or enhancing sexual connection.

The list above is not meant to be exhaustive but is intended to convey that the TCC process, infused with useful information, can be a vital adjunct to the counseling process. It is important for counselors to assess, be aware of possible skills deficits, and be open to exploring ways to remediate these issues. The needs will be as diverse as the methods for addressing these issues are. We encourage you to be creative and work with your clients to provide them with the most comprehensive care possible.

Step Seven: Termination

Termination in TCC follows the patterns commonly found in other counseling protocols. There is one obvious exception—the somewhat abstract idea that the counselor's relationship will no longer interact with the couple's relationship. Clients understand this by talking about couples they have known in the course of their lives together or even about their individual relationship with their parent's relationship during their formative years. We make this aspect of termination quite explicit by sharing openly how things might be different and encouraging the clients to realize the growth they have undergone through the course of their counseling. We also stress that relating to other couples, friends, and family can have profound positive effects for them as well as their counterparts. Few approaches prepare clients for the complexities of relating to other relationships as well as Tandem Counseling does.

We also tell couples that as they get close to termination, the potential for earlier problems to resurface increases. This causes some despair; the couple correctly assumed these problems had been resolved during the course of counseling and now their work seems to have come undone. In truth, fears of termination—of doing it on their own—and anxieties on how well the lessons will work, cause this eruption. By warning the couple early in the termination process, clients are not surprised when it happens and often treat it as a simple reality. The advanced notice actually encourages them to take what they have learned and rely upon the relationship to carry them through the uncertainty associated with termination. It's interesting to watch as clients help and support one another in ways they had previously never understood as they navigate the process of exiting therapy and moving forward as a couple.

Summary

TCC is a unique protocol for delivering couples counseling. In this chapter, we outlined the process of determining if a couple's referral for

TCC is warranted. We discussed how clients are seen separately for a brief course (4 to 8 weeks) of individual therapy and how the decision to move from individual to TCC is made. We differentiated the tandem counseling sessions by focusing on the ground rules and the special techniques that TCC employs. All these techniques capitalize on the fact that there are now two counselors in the room. Though this idea may be somewhat abstract to readers, we emphasized that with TCC, it is now possible for the counselor's relationship to play an active role in healing the clients' relationship.

The brief histories and examples of how we incorporated in vivo consultation, role-playing, and addressing skills deficits through imparting information, illustrate the steps we took to capitalize on a protocol that now placed four people in the counseling office instead of three. The work of Stan and Lacy provided some specific examples of how clients work to understand the concepts and experience this format differently from their previous traditional counseling efforts.

References

Anderson, S., Anderson, S., Palmer, K., Mutchler, M., & Baker, L. (2011). Defining high conflict. *American Journal of Family Therapy*, 39(1), 11–27.

Faber, A., & Mazlish, E. (2012). *How to talk so kids will listen and listen so kids will talk*. New York: Scribner.

Fall, K., & Howard, S. (2017). *Alternatives to domestic violence*. New York: Routledge.

Gottman, J. M., & Silver, N. (1999). *Seven principles for making marriage work*. New York: Three Rivers.

Lerner, H. (1997). *The dance of intimacy*. New York: Harper.

Nelson, J. (2006). *Positive discipline*. New York: Ballantine.

Siegel, D., & Bryson, T. (2016). *No drama discipline*. New York: Bantam.

6

TANDEM COUPLES COUNSELING WITH OTHER DYADS

The Adult Child-Parent Client

Chapter 5 provided an outline of the steps for facilitating a Tandem Couples Counseling (TCC) approach. In our own clinical work, married couples made up about 75% of the cases we saw in TCC. The other 25% consisted of different relational dyads, including adolescent siblings, parent and adolescent, business partners, and adult child and parent. The relationship dynamics varied for each but the TCC protocol remained consistent. We thought it would be helpful to explore the application of TCC with one of these unique pairings, so for this chapter, we will highlight the adult child and parent dyad.

Much of the literature on relationships between parents and their adult children are in the area of aging and parental death (Hagestad, 1984; 1987; King, 1993; Krause & Haverkamp, 1996; Lewis, 1990; Myers, 1988). The research literature demonstrates that the transition from a child-parent to an adult child-parent relationship is not always an easy one and the relationship expands in several ways as the parties get older. Relationships that adjust and evolve with the changing developmental phases tend to do better than those that adhere rigidly to relationship roles and norms. Helping people make healthy life transitions is an important part of counseling, so it makes sense that people in these relationships may seek assistance. The case presented in this chapter is one relationship that is struggling with the adult child and parent relationship. While this transition is a struggle for most, this case illustrates how historical fractures in the relationship can continue to create issues as the individuals get older, and the elements of high conflict can obstruct healthy development.

Case Study: William and Barton

This is the case of William and Barton. It provides an example of TCC applied to an adult child and parent dyad. It also illustrates a different pathway of entering TCC, rather than the more traditional route outlined in Chapter 5. As with the case of Stan and Lacy, the client material is used to illustrate the TCC approach and is not a verbatim account of the case.

Step One: Initial Contact

In this case, Barton was currently participating in individual counseling. During individual counseling, it became clear to the counselor that the relationship between Barton and his father was the primary area for growth. The idea for a joint meeting was explored in the following way:

Counselor: Barton, you have made quite a bit of progress in your intimate relationships, but it seems like we keep coming back to your relationship with your dad.

Barton: Yeah, I just can't shake it and it seems like no matter what I try, it doesn't get any better.

Counselor: What would you think about inviting your father in here, as a consultant to your process, for one or two sessions, to see if that produces some insight?

Barton: Well, he thinks counseling is for the weak (laughs), but he might like the consultant idea. He always was interested in ways to fix me.

Bringing the other person in as a consultant is a way to set clear boundaries about who is the client, but also provides a way to gain a distinct perspective on the relationship. In most cases, the plan would be for one or two sessions, and then back to the individual, but it can also uncover deeper issues that may be more appropriate for other forms of counseling.

Step Two: Intake and Assessment

The purpose of the conjoint sessions between William and Barton was to explore the relationship between the two more in-depth to catalyze the individual counseling of Barton. Here is what was learned about their relationship over the course of the two sessions.

William and Barton are father and son. William is a 64-year-old retired police officer and Barton is a 40-year-old salesman. William's wife—Barton's mother—Sylvia, died four years ago due to cancer. Barton reports that the relationship with his father has always been "tense," but the relationship has been worse since his mother's death. Barton had a three-year-old son, Riley, and Barton won't let William around Riley due to William's anger issues.

William presents as very controlled and agitated during the initial session. His perspective on the relationship is that Barton has always been "spoiled." William reports being gone a lot during Barton's early years and felt they never really connected. "Sylvia always babied him and when he acted up, that's when I come in. She's gone now and there's nothing I can do about that. Barton is just pissed that no one is around to cater to him."

Barton sees his dad as an angry, controlling person. He claims he doesn't really know his dad very well and never experienced the typical father-son bonding times that his friends had growing up. He resents how his dad criticizes him for having needs and rejects any attempt to connect as a sign of weakness. Barton believes his relationship with his father might be over. Barton is very protective of Riley and does not want to expose Riley to William, but also wants the relationship to improve because he is afraid he will turn out just like William. Attempts to reconcile have been failures, with much of the communication breaking down in the following way.

Counselor: Barton, tell me what you would like to happen with your relationship with your dad.

Barton:	I think I just want it to be better. I want to able to have him over for dinner. I want him to be able to babysit Riley, but all that seems so far away.
Counselor:	That's what you want to do, but what must change for that to happen?
Barton:	He needs to be nicer. He needs to stop being so critical and angry about everything. (William snorts).
Counselor:	What would you be willing to change?
Barton:	Me? Nothing. It's him that needs to change.
William:	Me? You are a sniveling little brat... good-for-nothin' ... this is such bullshit. Is that why you called me in her? To tell me I'm a bad person and call me names?
Counselor:	You are right, William. Our time is not best spent on name-calling. We are here to see what can be done to improve the relationship.
William:	It's him. It's always been him. Your mom pampered you and look at you now. She's gone and you are a wreck—can't even have a conversation without getting upset.
Barton:	This was a mistake. I'm leaving. (gets up and walks out).

Although the first session ended in Barton leaving, they both agreed to return for a second session. In the second session, a few things became clear. First, while Barton and William agreed that their history was unhealthy and conflicted, they did not agree on the reason for the disconnect. In short, Barton blamed William and William blamed Barton. This schism created an unscalable obstacle to change. The more the counselor explored one perspective, the farther away the other would move, feeling attacked, judged, and misunderstood. Second, it was clear that there was an enormous amount of pain embedded in the relationship. They both regretted the time lost and voiced a desire for a close relationship. Both have unresolved grief with their recent loss but are unable to utilize the relationship for healing.

Elements of High Conflict

Referring the dyad for further conjoint counseling is a possibility, but in consideration of utilizing TCC, an assessment of the conflict level of the dyad is appropriate. Barton and William report a conflict-based relationship for the duration of their relationship. When Baron left home at 18, he and William communicated through Sylvia. They got into a physical altercation at Sylvia's funeral and haven't spoken much since. The birth of Riley sparked renewed interest in developing the relationship but crumbled when Barton and William could not seem to be in contact without fighting and Barton made the decision to disconnect from William due to the conflict.

To assess high conflict, we will utilize a variety of elements noted in Chapter 2, drawn from Gottman and Silver (1999), Anderson, Anderson, Palmer, Mutchler, and Baker (2011), and our own experience. Gottman and Silver (1999) focused on married couples, but his elements of high conflict can be applied to this father and son dyad. When evaluating their communication patterns, there is evidence of an elevated level of all four elements—Criticism, Contempt, Defensiveness, and Stonewalling. They rate extremely high on the Criticism element, with both seeing the other as the primary cause of the relationship discord. William's perception of Barton as weak colors most of the interactions they have and has been a driving force in William's reason for cutting himself off from Barton. The contempt is evident; William notes, "Being around him makes me want to vomit sometimes. When he starts whining it just makes me sick." They both use Defensiveness as a primary relationship tool along with Stonewalling to keep the dysfunctional relationship dynamics in place. The starkest evidence of the presence of these elements rests in the fact that these two have not had any contact for several years and when they do, the interaction is volatile.

In examining William and Barton from Anderson et al.'s (2011) typology, there are considerable manifestations of both Clusters I: Pervasive Negative Exchanges and II: Hostile, Insecure, Emotional Environment. For Cluster I, the communication is predominantly, if not entirely, conflict-based. The two joint sessions were characterized by elevated levels of externalization, blaming, defensiveness, and hostility. Note the negativity in the choice of words and the change of flow when the counselor asks about positive aspects of the relationship and one another.

Counselor: We have talked quite a bit about what you would each like to change in the relationship. I am wondering about

	the parts that you would like to preserve. What are some things about the relationship that is worth holding on to? (silence)
Barton:	I guess I'll go. I think I would like to have a more normal father and son relationship. We never really had that. He was always at work or just away from home. He never did the normal stuff with me. It's like my childhood was ripped off.
William:	That's BS and you know it. I was trying to provide for you and your mother, and you just don't want to give me credit for that.
Counselor:	I want to interrupt here. I was asking about good things within the relationship and Barton; you gave me more of a wish of how you would like it to be. Can either of you identify one or two things that work within your relationship?
William:	If he would stand up and do something with his life, things would be better for everyone. I've tried to help you, but you don't seem to take to it. It's just more of the same with you.

For Cluster II, the relationship is marked by disconnect and withdrawal. When the two interact, the affective environment is permeated with a sense of tension and distrust. There is no willingness to be emotionally vulnerable, as both see the other person as unsafe. For most of the relationship, William and Barton relied on Sylvia to be the buffer. This relational pattern created an unhealthy triangle, which—although provided some protection from the conflict—prevented William and Barton from developing healthy ways of connecting and working through their issues. With Sylvia gone, the relationship has no way of coping and bridging the distance between them, so all that is left is the bitterness and fear.

Of the other factors of high conflict mentioned in Chapter 2, the only one that stands out is the Conflicting Family of Origin Patterns. This one is interesting because normally we are looking at how the couple's two separate families of origin norms and patterns clash as they form this new relationship. In the case of William and Barton, they shared a family of origin, so the assessment is about how that foundation was formed and the effects we are seeing echoed in the present-day relationship. If you think of a relationship as a house, and the family of origin patterns as the foundation, then experiencing cracks in that foundation can produce later structural issues in the house. In the case of William and Barton, the early years were characterized by distance and, from Barton's perspective, neglect. These patterns were not corrected over time and the relationship is experiencing the results of that shaky foundation in the present day.

Overall, it was felt that William and Barton would be appropriate for TCC intervention. The relationship has a long history of intense conflict which has evolved into the two not being able to be around or communicate with each other without volatile emotional or physical reactions. Although the birth of Barton's son has created a shift in motivation toward wanting to find a resolution, the high conflict patterns in the relationship could continue to interfere with the application of traditional conjoint counseling and the relationship modeling between the two counselors. The unique advantage of TCC was seen as a possible benefit to the dyad.

Step Three: The Transition to Individual Sessions

Once the dyad agreed to explore TCC, the decision-making about the individual counseling and choice of a counselor occurs collaboratively between clients and intake counselor. In this case, Barton already had a relationship with a counselor—who was also the counselor who conducted the temporary joint sessions—so it was decided that Barton would continue with it. That counselor made a referral to another counselor for William. In considering the dynamics and areas for growth within the relationship, the counselor reflected on the treatment goals and the potential quality of the co-therapy relationship when making the referral. In this case, Barton's counselor was an older male, working with a younger client, and he made a referral to a younger male counselor to work with William. The parallel process dynamics of this pairing will be discussed later. William met with the counselor and agreed to continue with the individual work with the goal of meeting again with Barton to continue the relationship work.

Step Four: Individual Sessions

As mentioned in Chapter 5, the tentative plan is to spend 4–8 weeks in individual counseling. During this time, the counselors will consult on a regular basis to focus on gaining insight into how the individual's movement fits into the larger relationship frame. This time will also be used by the co-therapists to develop the co-therapy relationship and think about how this relationship intersects with the rapport created with the clients in the individual work. It is this unique blend of relational attention that makes TCC different from traditional approaches.

The tasks associated with the individual sessions include:

1 Developing rapport between counselor and client;
2 Gaining insight into how intrapersonal issues have contributed to the relationship (both constructive and destructive); and
3 Building the skill at focusing on self and identifying at least one personal change he/she can bring to the relationship dynamic.

William in Individual Counseling

William had never attended counseling and his perception was that it was unnecessary, and that people use it as a crutch. He saw himself as an independent person who helped others—others did not help him. This allowed him to maintain a position of significance, and at times, control. Therefore, he approached individual counseling with caution and although building rapport with him was challenging, it underscored the importance of spending some time connecting with him, which built trust in the process and paved the way for vulnerability and growth. Through the therapeutic relationship, he experimented with the risks associated with trusting someone else and allowing them to provide care. Like many cases of high conflict relationships, the short amount of time in individual counseling provided a safe place to explore some of the underlying issues that the person did not feel safe enough to discuss within the relationship. When that type of paralysis occurs, the issue is just one part of the problem, while the additional problem becomes the inability to process it, and the dynamic of this obstruction creates a cycle that moves the relationship to an increasingly darker place. As William noted, "I didn't feel like I could talk to Barton about the death of his mom. The more time went by, the worse it became. Then I began to think he was a bad son for not talking about it or that I was a bad father for not talking about it. It just became this huge wall and it's so sad."

William also learned a great deal about how his way of life impacted his relationship with Barton. This move from external to an internal locus of control is a vital goal of the individual sessions, as the dedication to blame—a characteristic of high conflict couples—is one of the elements that make traditional forms of couples counseling so difficult. The following is just one example of how to begin this shift:

William: It just makes me so angry when Barton doesn't try hard enough. He just gives up.

Counselor: What do you see as your role when you perceive Barton giving up?

William: I'm his father, so I must stop him. I mean, what am I supposed to do, just let him give up without even trying?

Counselor: Maybe, I don't know. What I'm really interested in is what that looks like for you to "stop him."

William: Ummm ... I guess I tell him he's wrong, that he should try harder.

Counselor: So, you are trying to motivate him by using criticism.

William: Yeah, but as you say it, it sounds bad.

Counselor: What do you mean?

William: I don't like to think of myself as being critical, but I am. I never thought of it as a tool for motivating, but I do use it that way. I'm not sure if it works. My parents did that to me and I'm not sure if it ever worked for me either.

Counselor: How did you respond to your parents' attempts to motivate?

William: Hah! I fought them tooth and nail, but deep down inside it hurt. They were just doing the best they could.

> Counselor: So, it's possible that people such as yourself or your parents can have good intentions, like motivation, but produce some ineffective and even painful methods. What do you do when you know that's the case?
>
> William: You can change? Saying it aloud, it seems so simple. Just quit being such a jerk and maybe things would be different, better. I guess it's harder to do than say.

The forming of a trusting alliance with the counselor was a huge area of growth for William. As the sessions progressed, the gentle redirection from Barton's faults, to William's strengths and struggles, provided a focus on what William needed in his life and empowered him to center his efforts on the things he could control (his own thoughts, feelings, and behaviors) instead of elements he tries—but could not—control (the thought, feelings, and behaviors of others). Within these sessions, he moved away from blaming Barton and moved toward identifying ways he could make changes to improve the relationship. We firmly believe that, due to the elements of high conflict, William would have never been able to take the risk to focus on himself and be vulnerable and accountable within his relationship with Barton via traditional forms of couples counseling.

Barton in Individual Counseling

Much different from his father's expectations of counseling, Barton had positive experiences with individual counseling. He was accustomed to using counseling to explore relationship issues from his own perspective and was skilled at taking accountability for his change process but he hit a brick wall when trying to work through his relationship with his father. As the two conjoint sessions demonstrated, the dynamics in the relationship produced elevated levels of Barton's tendency to self-protect and withdraw from conflict. When in the presence of his father, he seemed incapable of accessing the strategies that served him so well in other relationships. Individual counseling allowed him time to regroup and refocus his efforts in a more productive manner.

While rapport building was easy for Barton, the tasks of focusing on self and identifying targets for personal change within the relationship with his father were more difficult for him. Patterns of his family origin, previously unexplored in his past counseling, became the focus of the sessions. The exploration unearthed an enormous amount of pain that had been buried by the safeguarding mechanisms of minimization and denial. There were several times in this process where Barton would pause and say, "I haven't thought about this in years. It's like I forgot it even happened" and begin to cry. The themes associated with these past events included feeling disconnected and uncared for by his father. He remembered one particularly painful moment when he was fifteen and had just broken up with his girlfriend. He worked up the courage to talk to his dad about it. He walked up to William and told him what happened, and tears began to form in his eyes. William responded, "Don't be such a pansy. I don't have time for this crap. I have to take a call." and walked out of the room, leaving Barton alone, crying. Barton said that typified his relationship with his dad and that he thinks he made a conscious choice at that moment, to sever his ties with his father.

Prior to the individual sessions, Barton viewed the problem as solely resting with William. This was calcified by Barton's refusal to talk or see his father for many years. When they would cross paths, the relationship would explode in pain and animosity, further maintaining the rigid rationale to disconnect. Meeting with William in the conjoint sessions served to stir up all the feelings and feed the perception that William rejected him and would never change. Barton used denial and minimization to push the issues away, but the feelings were still present and fueling the current intensity of the relational disconnect. The individual sessions helped facilitate the processing of these feelings, bringing them to the surface where they could be dealt with within the framework of individual choice.

Role of Co-therapy

TCC relies upon the ability of the counselors to relate to one another in an open and productive way, and therefore access the change potential of the co-therapy modality. As we mentioned earlier, the relationship between the counselors is used to gain deeper insight into the dyad's relationship and this insight, along with the implicit and explicit modeling of the co-therapy relationship, become agents of change with the TCC protocol. To ensure that the process honors this concern from the outset, both Barton and William review and sign releases allowing the counselors to discuss information obtained in the individual sessions. The information discussed focuses on two crucial elements:

1   How the intrapersonal impacts the interpersonal, and
2   How the information learned about the other client impacts the counselor.

If I am Barton's counselor, I would be listening to information about William through the lens of Barton. As I listen, I am paying attention to my thoughts and feelings about what I am hearing. These insights give me deeper information about Barton. I can then share those with my co-counselor and vice-versa. This process is vital and unique to TCC.

The parallel process occurs when the dynamics from one relationship carry over inconsistent relational patterns into another relationship. The parallel process concerns surface early in the TCC process. The client's themes and patterns of their relationship are reflected within the counselors and their relationship as they consult with one another. We learned to fully appreciate the value of these dynamics in our consultative relationship because they completely illuminate the struggles the clients' experience and highlight the important utility of the co-therapy relationship—an aspect routinely ignored by many who use co-therapy.

For example, during consultation meetings, Barton's counselor, echoing his client's patterns, noticed an urge or tendency to want to withdraw as William's counselor voiced frustration about the lack of progress in Barton's individual work. When counselors expect parallel process effects to surface, they work through the biases brought on by the influence of their respective clients and craft an approach that more accurately honors their client's struggles. The journey can be perilous if counselors ignore the parallel process effects. Unhealthy triangulations where the counselors and clients unite against each other severely inhibit the process. On the other hand, when these patterns are discussed rather than "acted out," clients obtain valuable insights about their relationship and they identify points where strengthening is possible. The next examples provide another glimpse into the role of the co-therapy relationship and how it manages and uses a parallel process.

Co-counselor Consult #1

This consult occurred after the first individual session. The counselors decided to meet early in the process due to William's extreme distrust of counseling.

Counselor 1:   Thanks for meeting with me. I met with William and it went surprisingly well. Perhaps I can give you my take on the session and we can go from there? You can listen and give me Barton's perspective on whatever comes up.

Counselor 2:   That sounds great.

Counselor 1:   Okay, well, William was a bit hesitant about counseling. I let him talk about that for a while and he also mentioned, by way of example, that Barton had been in therapy forever and it didn't seem to do him any good.

Counselor 2:   Interesting.

Counselor 1:   We did manage to explore a bit of his family of origin, which sounded grim. I think he worries about Barton a lot and just feels like every attempt he makes causes Barton to either roll up in a ball or run away.

Counselor 2:   Uh-huh.

Counselor 1:   He had several examples of how he has tried to make contact over the years but claims nothing really makes a difference. I didn't get a sense of how he would like to change his approach. We aren't there yet, and right now I think he firmly believes that Barton is the largest obstacle to their relationship.

Counselor 2:   Yeah...

Counselor 1:   I noticed you are pretty quiet. How are you doing with what I am sharing?

Counselor 2:   Wow, you know, I was just taking it all in and trying to hear you as Barton might and I just felt really discouraged. I felt blamed and a bit hopeless about the prospect of change. I think that it's a pretty clean read on how Barton must feel.

Counselor 1:   That's actually good in my opinion. That's what we are using these consultations for—to try to get a richer sense of where our clients are coming from within the relationship. It sounds like this validates some of the dynamics that the clients have been reporting and we can take this back to our individual sessions and use it to build rapport and eventually move towards change.

Co-counselor Consult #2

The consult was conducted after the fifth session.

Counselor 2:   Okay, nice to see you again. Barton is making some substantial progress in the individual sessions. I would like to hear how William is doing, and maybe get a sense of how far away we are from meeting together.

Counselor 1:   Sounds good. I think William is breaking through some of the protective layers he has built up over the years and is beginning to gain insight into what is underneath. He has talked about the fear of connecting and the pain of feeling alone.

Counselor 2:   That sounds good. I think Barton would be surprised to hear that there is anything behind the anger or criticism. Well, maybe that's not 100% true. I think he might guess there is something back there but would think William would never admit it.

Counselor 1:   The protective layers keep people from expecting a more sensitive side.

Counselor 2:   Would you be willing to talk as William and just explain that a bit more? I want to see what that would feel like from Barton's perspective.

Counselor 1:   Sure. I am afraid that if people know about my sensitive side, they will see me as weak and take advantage of me or even hurt me. I think that's why

	I am so hard on you. I don't hate you; I'm not disappointed in you. I just don't want you to get hurt.
Counselor 2:	Barton would be blown away if he heard that from his dad. As I'm listening, I don't have the slightest urge to disconnect. I don't feel attacked. If anything, I feel like I want to know more.
Counselor 1:	I think one more session and William will be more confident in sharing these aspects of self. It has been a lot for him to trust, but I think he likes it. Let's touch base next week and see if we want to transition to joint sessions.

Step Five: Dyad is Readied for Joint Sessions

The individual sessions help clients identify the personal issues that may be adversely affecting their relationship, support them as they unearth concerns, move from an external focus to a more internal focus, develop plans for change, and identify resources that will be helpful to their personal efforts and their relationship. This explicit relationship focus differentiates TCC preliminary individual counseling from individual counseling in general. Within the relatively safe individual sessions, clients gain insights about how their patterns impact their perspective of the relationship. They begin to realize how easily they misunderstand or misinterpret one another and how much energy it takes to correct their assumptions. We confirm these changes by directly observing the client as they correctly surmise the impact their patterns and initiated discussions have on their relationship and with others who participate in the pattern.

In TCC, planning for the joint sessions begins at the onset of the individual work. Each counselor develops hypotheses about their client and the relationship, and these insights are shared via consultations that invite the counselors to discuss their findings and refine their assumptions about the dyad's struggles and resources. Removed from the obstacles created by the high conflict that intensify in conjoint sessions, individual sessions produce a wealth of valuable information about each person, enabling counselors to quickly identify the relationship themes and patterns of interaction. Armed with this information, counselors better anticipate where conflicts arise, how misunderstanding occurs, the effects of each person's history on the relationship, and possible directions to pursue the connection to successfully replace conflict.

As the counselors begin to sense that the individuals are ready to meet jointly, this potential for transition is discussed with each client. It is typical for this discussion to produce some anxiety in the clients. Fear of being ready and moving out of the comfort of the individual sessions and into the unknown of the joint sessions are typical topics for exploration. Keep in mind that each client is perceiving the potential joint counseling based on their past experiences of failure and conflict, so it is normal for them to be apprehensive. With TCC, the advantage is that each client is bringing with them a counselor who has conveyed an understanding of them at a deep level. With a connection established, there is no longer any need to compete to convince the third party (counselor) that any personal position is the correct one. Reflecting on the work accomplished in the individual sessions can replace the overriding fear with hope about the upcoming conjoint sessions.

With the gains made in the individual session and a sense of connection with a counselor, the entry into the joint session will noticeably be different from previous experiences with counseling. Instead of beginning the work full of apprehension and high conflict, each client now possesses the option to express what they have learned about themselves and how it impacts the relationship. Even more importantly, each person will identify what they can change to produce a different outcome. This is vastly different from the typical, "I am not getting my needs met and this is what you can do differently" dynamic that represents the start of other forms of relational therapy.

Step Six: Tandem Sessions

As the dyad readies for work in tandem sessions, we outline the basic goals and rules to avoid any confusion and to help them settle into the pattern that will form the remainder of their therapy. This dyad is unique from many of the married couples we had worked with as this has not spoken to each other for quite some time. If fact, the first joint session—when William was brought in as a consultant for Barton's individual counseling—was the first time they had participated in a meaningful conversation in years. While the individual sessions are designed to break away some of the obstacles and pave a way to connect, there will still be some anxiety and the danger of old patterns flooding the tandem sessions. To set the stage for the tandem work, we orient them to the process.

We remind them that all our efforts will be focused on helping to understand their relationship and to implement better ways of becoming responsible stewards of that relationship. We remind them that in the tandem sessions there are no restrictions on patterns of interaction—counselors and clients are free to speak and offer questions to anyone they choose. While the individual sessions were conducted with one counselor and one, client the tandem sessions open a range of interactions within what is now a small group.

In choosing co-therapists, the initial counselor specifically chose a younger male to work with William. With this setup, the co-therapists uniquely mirrored the age of the clients. This allowed a couple of interesting processing possibilities. Primarily, it gave each client an advocate similar in age from the other pair. During the individual sessions, it allowed each to work through some of the issues of trust and connection as the therapeutic relationship was developed. In a sense, the therapeutic relationship became a test run for what the process could look like moving forward. As the work moved to the tandem sessions, the co-therapists were free to make use of this dynamic in their roles plays and in vivo consultations.

Stress a Focus on the Relationship

In the tandem sessions, the dyad understands that the primary goal is to improve the relationship. Now that they each have insight into the relationship patterns and have generated ideas for change, we encouraged them to think before they act and to ask, "Does this action improve, have no impact on, or hurt the relationship?" This question can also be used as an assessment for choices made and helps avoid drifting back to individual needs and concerns. Here is one exchange where this relational assessment process was used.

Counselor 1:   So, you mentioned that you tried to meet for lunch this week. I'm wondering how that went.

Barton: Yeah, I thought it would be a good idea to try some of the things out that we have been working on here. It was like a test to see if we could do it without you two (laughs).

Counselor 2:   Yes, being able to translate what we do in here to the outside world is important. William, what was your thought about the lunch idea?

William: I thought it was a good idea. I was a bit nervous, but we did it anyway.

Counselor 2:   I'm curious, did you talk to Barton about being anxious?

William: Ha! I knew you would ask that question. At first, I was going to keep quiet, but I had your voice in my head saying, "That's the old pattern, William." So, I thought about it and tried to ask myself if talking about it was good or bad for the relationship. It made me uncomfortable, but I thought it would be good for a relationship, to be honest, and not try to protect myself or Barton from my feelings. So, I told him.

Counselor 1:   Great use of the assessment!

Barton: I was shocked at first when he told me, and I felt myself wanting to just call it off. I heard his anxiety as an attack like I was making him anxious. But I caught myself and realized I was feeling nervous about it myself. So, I was able to say, "Me, too!" and then we laughed and moved forward.

Counselor 1:   It's a nice example of how considering what the relationship needs can move you past your old patterns and into more connected ways of being. That pathway is not without risk—I mean you still had anxiety—but it provided you with a relational way to deal with it.

In Vivo Consultations

The joint sessions allow the co-therapist consultations to occur in the present and presence of the clients. This process is unique to TCC when combined with the individual sessions and the ways the co-therapy relationship is utilized. While there may be some models that make use of co-therapy from time to time, TCC is unique in its focus on the co-therapy relationship as an agent of change. By purposefully using co-therapy this way, we provide insight into the inter and intrapersonal patterns of our clients in an immediate way and model cooperation and other related skills in the way we communicate with each other during the consultation.

In vivo consultations can also be used to broach subjects that are rigidly avoided by the clients. The consultation can be a way to start the conversation and model how the processing of these painful experiences can be handled in a healthy way. In the case of William and Barton, the death of Sylvia was one of those issues not being discussed within the relationship. Both counselors had explored it during the individual sessions, so they each had a clear sense of how their clients were perceiving the issue. The old pattern remained during the joint sessions, and in vivo consultation was used to break it.

Barton:	I guess there are some things that can't be undone. Things we just can't repair.
Counselor: 1:	What are some of those things? I'm uncertain about what you mean.
Barton:	I don't really know. You know, past stuff. I don't know. I shouldn't be bringing this stuff up. I should be happy we are making progress. I don't know why I must do that.
Counselor 1:	I think I want to consult with Counselor 2 for a minute.
Counselor 2:	What are you hearing?
Counselor 1:	I am noticing that Barton is getting very vague, but it also thinking about something that I think is important to him. Listening to his struggle, Sylvia comes to mind.

Counselor 2:   Hmmm... yes, she is on my mind too. When I listen to Barton through William's perspective, I hear him struggling and I want Sylvia to appear and comfort him. I am very aware, in those moments, how much she is missed by both.

Counselor 1:   Yes, her death created a lack of comfort in this relationship. It is encouraging them to provide each other of it, instead of relying on her. But experiencing that void also reminds them that she is gone, but they aren't talking about that. The old pattern is to fear the discomfort and not trust the relationship to deal with it. When it surfaces, Barton wants to run, and William gets prickly.

Counselor 2:   Maybe it's time we did talk about what they want to do differently with this aspect of their lives that is producing so much fear and pain.

In this example, the in vivo consultation is used to address the issue of the death of Sylvia and bring those issues to a place they can be discussed openly. This process is more effective because it weaves the presenting issue into other patterns and elements that have been at the core of the work, which makes the clients less defensive. The processing between the co-therapists also provides a direct yet gentle invitation to the clients to join the discussion and creates more flow than in traditional forms of counseling. In other words, it is impossible to have this sort of process observation intervention with only one counselor. To do so, you would have to make the process observation solo—directly to the clients—which would have a greater chance of triggering their conflict responses. Utilizing co-therapy in this way provides a readily available advantage is this arena.

In vivo consultations can also be used to model skills pertinent to the clients. We like to use the consultations early as ways to demonstrate the skills in a passive, perhaps covert, way but this technique can also be used in later sessions to illustrate skills that the clients may be struggling to replicate. Conflict management and healthy disagreement are always good candidates for modeling, as high conflict relationships tend to wrestle with these the most. In this example, disagreement is modeled.

You will notice that the skill is not explicitly stated before the consultation, so we do not say, "We are now going to model healthy disagreement." Instead, the skill is embedded in the communication within the consultation and the clients are merely exposed, they can then be processed after consultation to assess what the clients observed.

Counselor 2: I need a moment to consult with Counselor 1.

Counselor 1: I am ready.

Counselor 2: As I was listening to the last exchange between you and Barton, I was noticing that I was getting increasingly restless. I am trying to locate what exactly was bothering me so much.

Counselor 1: Hmm ... well, we were exploring Barton's feelings of disconnect in a wide variety of relationships.

Counselor 2: Yes, I tracked that. At some point in the conversation, I started to feel that Barton was moving out of the center of the discussion—like the disconnect is caused by others and Barton is the victim. Yes, that's it.

Counselor 1: Okay, so you felt like the conversation was lacking in accountability.

Counselor 2: Yes, now that I have had time to think about it, that is it exactly. I felt like Barton was not taking responsibility for his part in those disconnects.

Counselor 1: And you are probably frustrated that I wasn't doing anything about it.

Counselor 2: Yes, that is why I wanted to talk about it. I wanted to address it openly instead of stewing about it or jumping in and acting out in frustration.

Counselor 1: I see where you are coming from. I think I had a handle on it, but I was taking a long way home (laughs).

Counselor 2: That makes sense. I trust you know what you are doing, but also want to know that I can share what I am seeing.

Counselor 1: Absolutely.

In this example, the counselors were able to model some healthy disagreement skills. Counselor 2 was able to share feelings openly instead of attacking (William) or withdrawing (Barton). Counselor 1 demonstrated open listening and conveyed understanding without being overly apologetic or taking responsibility for something he felt he didn't do. There was no name-calling, shaming, blaming, or walking out—strategies common to William and Barton. After the consultation, the group could process what occurred and themes could be highlighted.

Role-Playing

While the in vivo consultations are the best example of how to utilize the co-therapy relationship in TCC, the use of role-playing by the counselors is another unique facet of the approach. The in-depth knowledge of the client gained in the individual sessions provides each counselor with a focused sense of their client's motivations and patterns. At any point in the process, the counselors can act out a relational interaction, providing the clients with another vantage point to experience their dynamics. It is also possible for the clients to request a role-play to better understand a complex interpersonal interchange. We believe this additional perspective and experience allows the clients to move above the conflict and still be engaged in the process. In the case of William and Barton, where the two had been disconnected for so long, the role-playing was instrumental in getting them involved in some of the deeper issues in a gradual and less defended manner.

In many instances, role-playing is initiated when the counselors are sensing confusion or stonewalling while exploring an issue or dynamic. Role-playing can then be used to act as a defense eroding catalyst as illustrated below.

Barton:	I guess I just don't get what you are saying about the purpose or benefit of vulnerability. I get in in theory but don't see how that would ever work for us.
Counselor 1:	You are apprehensive about being vulnerable to William. You don't feel safe.

Barton:	Yeah, and that feeling just makes me not even want to try.
Counselor 1:	Okay, well why don't we show you what the differences look like between being vulnerable and guarded. We will act out both scenarios and get your feedback. As your counselor, I will play as you and Counselor 2 will be William.
Counselor 1 (Barton):	Dad, Riley's birthday is coming up and I would like you to be able to come over.
Counselor 2 (William):	That's nice. Am I allowed to be there? What does "to be able to come over" mean?
Counselor 1:	It means I need to be sure you are going to behave yourself when you come over.
Counselor 2:	What the hell does that mean? Who are you to tell me how to behave? Why don't you worry about your own stuff and quit starting stuff with me?
Counselor 1:	Fine, I knew it was a bad idea to even ask. <End role play>
Counselor 1:	Okay, what's your thought on that, specifically with regards to vulnerability?
Barton:	(laughs) I think we've had this exact conversation. I think this is how we do it. It doesn't seem vulnerable at all and we both walk away feeling bad.
William:	When it goes down like that, I feel bad, but at the same time, if that's how it's going to be, I don't really want to be around him. Like you acted out, I do tend to cue on certain words to try to get a sense of where he's coming from, but to be honest, I tend to assume he's going to blame me for something right from the beginning.
Counselor 2:	Okay, great. So, you recognize the old pattern and have some understanding that

	it is not working for you. It protects you but does not help improve the relationship. So, let's try a different way with the same discussion.
Counselor 1 (Barton):	Dad, Riley's birthday coming up and I would like you to be able to come over.
Counselor 2 (William):	I would really like to be there. It sounds fun!
Counselor 1 (Barton):	I am a little worried about how our relationship might impact the event. I don't want us to fight. I know it's not all you; I'm just putting it out there as a concern.
Counselor 2 (William):	I don't want to fight either, so I understand your worry. Maybe we can help each other stay on the right path, agree to step away from the party, like halfway through, and check-in with one another? Try to catch any issues early?
Counselor 1 (Barton):	That's a great idea. We can focus on enjoying the party and address any concerns at the midpoint. Can we also be in contact at the end of the evening to talk about how it all went?
Counselor 2 (William):	Sure. <End role play>
Counselor 1:	Okay, thoughts?
William:	That was a lot better. I have to admit, I still got tense after your first sentence.
Counselor 2:	What did you notice in my response? What did I focus on?
William:	Well, you bypassed all the possible traps, the negative perceptions I might have had about certain words. You just focused on how you felt about the core of the statement, which was being invited to a party.

Counselor 1:	Nice observation! Barton, what did you notice?
Barton:	I liked how you (I) was able to stay with the concern and try to voice what I was worried about but in a nonattacking way—I didn't back down, but I also wasn't making my point by being aggressive. I also didn't really focus on him; I tried to share the concern.
William:	And it was almost like you (I) was able to stay focused and work towards finding a way to address his worry and move to get to do what I wanted to do—which was to go to the party! I think a lot of times, I lose that focus and end up fighting, and, in the end, I might win but I lose the primary goal.
Counselor:	And all that was achieved through vulnerability—staying connected even when things get uncomfortable.

Information Sharing

This aspect of TCC was not utilized too extensively with this dyad. With William and Barton, learning ways of reconnecting and re-establishing their relationship was the primary goal. Skills deficits related to this goal were more easily ameliorated within the structure of TCC than in their previous attempts to remediate their issues.

One area in need of attention was with grief. The death of Sylvia impacted both William and Barton in significant ways and their relationship was too conflicted to provide space for healing. With the knowledge they gained in TTC, both Barton and William were able to fully explore her death—both individually and together. William asked for suggestions for reading material on grief and Barton later asked for information related to referrals for grief groups. Both avenues produced valuable pathways for growth that had previously been obstructed and denied by the conflict in the relationship.

Step Seven: Termination

As with other forms of counseling, under ideal circumstances, termination is a process that occurs when the clients have reached their goals. For William and Barton, termination was discussed once each client had good insight into their intrapersonal dynamics, understood how these dynamics manifested in their interpersonal relationships and began to take steps to change the relationship in positive ways.

For William, this meant understanding how his family of origin experiences had shaped his protective yet distant approach to his son. He gained some empathy-based awareness of how his patterns impacted his son and moved away from blaming Barton and began to think about how he could make changes in his connections to people. In many ways, this change was realized the more he was open and honest with Barton, sharing a wide continuum of feelings and thoughts. The more he experimented with honesty and transparency, the more vulnerable he felt. Instead of retreating to old patterns when confronted with those difficult emotions, he leaned into the relationship. This process did not always have positive results, but with each attempt, William became more confident in his new developing approach regardless of the outcome.

Barton made great strides in being courageous when he really wanted to withdraw. He began to understand that if a connection was desired, then he would need to take risks—even when confronted with information, feedback, or feelings he didn't like. The loss of his mother meant the loss of his main comforter in life. He made a choice to go out and create a relationship that provided a sense of nurturing for him, but he also decided to try to be comforting to others as well. He took steps to insert comfort into his relationship with his father, —something that had never been present in that relationship.

Summary

In this chapter, we explored the application of TCC with a relationship different from a traditional married couple. Although the dynamics were different, the application of the approach followed the same protocol. The presence of high conflict dynamics was problematic to the application of other forms of counseling, and the unique elements of TCC posed practical solutions to the clients' presenting issues.

References

Anderson, S., Anderson, S., Palmer, K., Mutchler, M., & Baker, L. (2011). Defining high conflict. *American Journal of Family Therapy*, 39(1), 11–27.

Gottman, J. M., & Silver, N. (1999). *Seven principles for making marriage work*. New York: Three Rivers.

Hagestad, G. O. (1984). The continuous bond: A dynamic, multi-generational perspective on parent-child relations between adults. In M. Perlmutter (Ed.), *Parent-child interaction and parent-child relations in child development* (pp. 129–158). Hillsdale, NJ: Erlbaum.

Hagestad, G. O. (1987). Parent-child relations in later life: Trends and gaps in past research. In J. B. Lancaster, J. Altmann, A. S. Rossi & L. R. Sherrod (Eds.), *Parenting across the life span: Biosocial dimensions* (pp. 405–433). New York: Aldine de Gruyter.

King, T. (1993). The experiences of midlife daughters who are caregivers for their mothers. *Health Care for Women International*, 14, 419–426.

Krause, A. M., & Haverkamp, B. E. (1996). Attachment in adult child-older parent relationships: Research, theory, and practice. *Journal of Counseling & Development*, 75(2), 83–92.

Lewis, R. A. (1990). The adult child and older parents. In T. H. Brubaker (Ed.), *Family relationships in later life* (pp. 68–85). Newbury Park, CA: Sage.

Myers, J. E. (1988). The mid/late life generation gap: Adult children with aging parents. *Journal of Counseling & Development*, 66(7), 331–335.

7

CONSULTATION AND SUPERVISION WITHIN TANDEM COUPLES COUNSELING

Unfortunately, while co-therapy is widely used in training centers, many—if not most—fail to reap the full benefits of the co-therapy relationship. This is not only regarding the practice but also with supervision. In many cases, the supervisors are not fully aware of the co-therapy clinical rationale and use it only for convenience. This chapter will outline a process of using Tandem Couples Counseling (TCC) philosophy and practice to augment existing training experiences in terms of co-therapist consultation and supervision. Examples will be given on how to oversee tandem teams and how to best use practices from the fields of group work and clinical supervision to enhance the depth of co-therapy. Common pitfalls arising in the process will also be highlighted with accompanying supervision strategies for prevention and remediation.

While TCC offers a novel protocol for delivering couples counseling, it also demands the same rugged adherence to effective supervision and consultation methods found in any form of counseling. There may be some differences in how supervision and consultation are delivered, but the need for both is significant. In this chapter, we discuss how to use supervision as a TCC counselor and include information on how to conduct the supervision of TCC counselors in your own practice.

Preparing for Consultation and Supervision in TCC

All supervision and consultation efforts are focused on three main goals:

1 Facilitation of counselor professional and personal development;
2 Promotion of counseling competencies; and
3 Promotion of accountable counseling services and programs (Bradley, Ladany, Hendricks, Whiting, & Rhode, 2010, p. 6).

The single difference between supervision and consultation lies in responsibility. In supervision, the *supervisor* is responsible for the actions of the counselor; in consultation, the *counselor* is solely responsible. Most general models of consultation-supervision will work effectively with TCC counselors if the therapist pair's relationship and efficacy are continuously addressed and assessed as a tool to help the couple. The most common models include (1) developmental, (2) integrated, and (3) orientation specific. Abundant supervision literature exists to help supervisors or consultants decide which model to select based on the experience levels of counselors and the type of clients served. In addition to these general concerns, TCC requires supervisors and consultants to invest a generous portion of supervision time in the counselor's relationship. With so many high-grade, readily available supervision texts, we opted to concentrate on the critical co-therapy elements of supervision and consultation in this chapter.

The adage, "It's the relationship that heals" is as true in TCC as in any other counseling situation. However, the saying takes on new meaning in the context of TCC; it should more appropriately read, "It is the relationship between the counselors that heals the couple's relationship." The idea may be a bit abstract but it is not invalid; TCC capitalizes on how effectively the two relationships work together to resolve conflict, improve intimacy, and resolve family of origin issues in compassionate and understanding ways. This unique clinical reality places a heavy burden on counselors who wish to conduct TCC sessions. Such counselors need not only be well-trained but also cultivate and maintain a strong relationship with another clinician who can effectively cooperate as a team to improve the relationship of the clients they are working. When the relationship is acting as an agent of change, there will be times when disagreements occur. TCC can produce a good deal of stress on the counselor's relationship—and their willingness to manage that stress openly and effectively makes a stark difference in the effectiveness of the counseling enterprise. In fact, when working with high conflict couples with the awareness and desired cultivation of a parallel process, conflict between counselors is expected and has potential value in the couple's treatment. However, there are times when conflict becomes an obstacle, and outside supervision is encouraged during these times. In our practice, TCC seemed to operate as Triadic Couples Counseling, as we liberally used the supervision of an outside colleague to provide feedback on the process.

While a traditional supervisor will consistently ask about the therapeutic relationship, the therapeutic relationship is defined more broadly in TCC. In this setting, the relationship between the counselors is as important as the relationship between the therapists and the couple. To be more precise, the supervisor or consultant must manage a critical, but abstract, reality: the relationship between the counselors interacts with (and hopefully aids) the relationship between the couple. To help clarify the point, we'll ask you to think about any couple you have a history with. When you think about that couple, you can easily separate and think of how you feel about them individually but it is also possible to recognize the entity that emerges from their relationship—a kind of "third person"—that is the amalgam of the two. It is exactly that "third person" emerging from the TCC counseling pair that must be addressed during any TCC supervision or consultation. The counselors need to be aware of the third entity, how the client couple is perceiving it, and how it can be improved and nurtured to increase effectiveness. This goal is one of the more important tasks that supervisors and consultants deal with as they help the counselors manage a list of interpersonal characteristics that are necessary precursors of the relationship that TCC counselors seek to offer to their clients.

To help guide the TCC counselor in the supervision and the consultation process, we usually ask the counselor to focus on self and the relationship, via the mindfulness process discussed in Chapter 4. We also find it helpful to monitor skill development. The following TCC Counselors' Skills in Table 7.1 lists the elements supervisors and consultants will need to address regarding the counselor pair.

Table 7.1 TCC Counselors' Skills.

Category	Item	Description
Relational		
	Respect	Ability to honor one another's opinions and ideas.
	Cooperation	Working together in the care of the couple.
	Integrity	Ability to deal with one another and the couple honestly and accurately.
	Accountability	Individual ownership of results and actions.
	Responsibility	Completing tasks and meeting expectations cooperatively.
	Intimacy	Ability to recognize, manage, and cultivate emotional intimacy effectively.
	Vulnerability	Openness to and acceptance of clients and co-counselor.
Clinical-Theoretical		
	Theoretical	How well conceptualizations interlace.
	Treatment	Collaborative interventions and assessments.
	Effectiveness	Continuous assessments of methods, interventions, and clinical relationships.
	Ethical Concerns	Continuous attention to ethical issues and their resolution.
Clinical-Practice		
	Role-Playing	Effectively assuming and acting out client roles and interactions.
	In Vivo Consultation	Consulting with the other counselor in front of the clients and processing their reactions.
	Modeling	Illustrating adaptive ways of managing differences of opinion, dealing with fears, etc.
	Boundaries	Cooperatively agreeing to and establishing proper limits and boundaries.
	Risk Assessments	Cooperatively evaluate risk and benefits for select interventions and client concerns.
	Peer Consultation-Supervision	Allocating the proper amount of time to regularly meet and discuss the course of the therapy and attend to critical elements of the counselors' relationship.

With a firm foundation to reflect on self, the relationship, and the necessary skills, we believe counselors will be prepared to make the most of consultations and supervision. It's not surprising that the co-therapy issues to be addressed are the same for any couple. For example, the relational skills listed in the TCC Counselor Checklist could just as easily be applied to guide any couple wanting to cooperate. This section is organized around five different problem areas. The following four potential problem areas were drawn from Roller and Nelson's, "The Five C's of Co-therapy that Delimit Effectiveness" (1991, p. 100): (a) Competition, (b) Confusion or Lack of Communication, (c) Lack of Congruence, and (d) Countertransference between the counselors. To this list, we add Parallel Process as the fifth source of problems. These potential hazards require continuous attention to ensure that TCC counselors provide the proper clinical relationship to their clients. We include them in this chapter because we have found that it is within the consultation-supervision process that these issues can be identified, explored, and reforged from problems to potential benefits within the couple's counseling.

Competition can quickly tarnish any relationship because it rapidly leads to resentments. It usually surfaces as a need to be right, to be better than, or to garner more attention. Unfortunately, competition is often based upon fears that are not easily identifiable, so supervisors and consultants need to be particularly astute and thorough. As a counselor preparing oneself for consultation and supervision, it is a good idea to consider your personal way of noticing if the competition is affecting a working relationship and if the tools used for managing competition are effective. The key insight is focused on identifying your pattern of competition and then discussing that pattern with your co-therapy partner. We stress the importance of recognizing this pattern because of the seriousness of a clinical situation where a competing couple is exposed to competing therapists. The fears within the couple and the counselors not being effectively managed—and acting out in the form of competition—can only produce undesired outcomes. In this case, rapid identification and correction are vital.

Consider a situation where a highly competitive couple enters counseling because of increased strife in their marriage. They report that they consistently try to best one another in everything—tennis matches have become so serious that they decided not to play together at all. They compete over their kids' affection, friends, income, and how much time they spend with one another's extended families. They entered TCC because of a referral from their traditional couple's counselor. After several months, the couple had made almost no progress, so they decided to try TCC hoping that it might be more effective.

One of their TCC counselors had been in practice for years and his reputation was well known in the community. His partner was younger and only in practice for a few years. The first TCC session went well according to the experienced counselor, contrary to what his co-therapist claimed. According to the less experienced counselor, the couple consistently deferred to the older counselor and acted like he was not in the room. When this perception was shared with the more experienced counselor, he responded by saying he did not experience that at all—the couple was simply more comfortable and interested in what he had to say. The counselors had previously experienced differences of opinion, but they had been quickly and easily resolved in past situations. This problem was different because there seemed no point of connection; they were seeing two vastly different things as they sat in the same session.

When encountering significant differences these counselors regularly pursued supervision, so they scheduled a meeting with a colleague who was knowledgeable about TCC. The consultant was impressed by how different their experiences were and began to ask questions about each counselor's views, but that strategy further frustrated them. The supervisor asked how these clients were affecting their professional relationship. The less experienced counselor maintained that he felt unimportant, even useless, at times; the more experienced counselor felt very flattered and enthusiastic. "So," the supervisor said, "it seems that one of you is winning and the other is losing, correct?" Sadly, he added, "In this situation, you cannot be model partners, you can only be one up and one down." The counselors' odd expressions on their faces convinced the supervisor that his point had its desired impact. The counselors could now realize how quickly and subliminally the clients' competitive difficulties "infected" their own relationship. The simple act of paying attention to only one counselor allowed a competitive process to surface without the couple uttering a word. It took almost no time to develop a good strategy for the in vivo consultation in the next session with the couple. It also helped the experienced counselor to admit the flattery made it difficult for him to see what exactly was going on. The less experienced counselor countered with his own understanding of how easily he can fall into a "victim role." These insights played a significant role in restoring the counselors' relationship, and the process helped both counselors understand what it's like to be the couple—or interact with them.

Confusion and lack of communication are two of the most identified couples' problems. In fact, most couples who come to therapy will tell you—without any prompting—that they are there due to "communication problems." It is obvious that TCC counselors need to be highly skilled communicators with and of themselves, and with their clients. This takes time and commitment on both parts. It is one of the reasons that TCC counselors must agree to meet and consult with one another outside of the regular counseling sessions. Clients look to counselors for a respectful and effective model of communication and expect their counselors to demonstrate useful ways of managing confusion and uncertainty. Many couples experience the ill effect chaos has in their lives, so anytime a counselor increases confusion or inhibits communication, the clients suffer greatly.

In TCC—confusion and its graver relative, chaos—are common issues. Many people who struggle in relationships have life histories that were deep and negative, contributing to the confusion and chaos in their families and lives. Communication problems are intricately linked to confusion because difficulty in communicating creates uncertainty. The most common reaction to confusion, chaos, and persistent communication problems is always some level of fear. Unfortunately, as we previously illustrated, anger is the preferred way people express their fear to others. So very often, people sense their anger but cannot articulate the fear that propels it. Under these circumstances, communication problems and confusion affecting counselors can have devastating effects. Clients come to counseling to reduce fears—try to make life less chaotic—and learn to share their thoughts and feelings more openly and effectively, so intimacy can flourish within their relationship. Effective counselors would do everything in their power to help achieve these goals.

Counselors are human beings, and under certain circumstances, they could interact in unclear ways, increase uncertainty, and inadvertently elevate fear in the couple and the process. Counselors will tend to react in unproductive ways when they are fearful. Fortunately, there are two people in the counseling session, and TCC can manage and contain fear and anxiety more effectively than traditional settings. Confusing comments or potentially chaotic situations are more easily handled using TCC methods like role-playing and in vivo consultations. TCC better mitigating such effects is no reason to ignore the potential; communication issues and confusion should always be on the counselors', supervisors', and consultants' agenda.

Despite TCC's advantages, there are times when a counselor's fear can affect the session by creating confusion and interrupting the established pattern of communication. An interesting example can be found in the use of individual sessions to augment the couple's sessions. Recall that by using TCC methods, a particular counselor can meet with his or her client in individual sessions as deemed necessary. This interesting option is not possible in traditional couples counseling because of the adverse triangulation effects that come from one counselor meeting privately with one member of the couple. How the decision to meet separately is made is as important as the reason to do so.

During a TCC counseling session with a high-conflict couple, one of the counselors announced that he would be meeting with the wife in an individual session between the current session and the next scheduled couple's session. The announcement came without the benefit of discussion among the foursome. The tension emanating from the unilateral decision was palpable, and the other counselor was clearly confused and worried that the sudden decision would harm their efforts to help the couple. In high-conflict couples, such communication problems usually spawn intense reactions and suspicion. Fortunately, the counselor who announced the decision immediately backtracked and asked for time to discuss the concerns he wanted to raise in the proposed individual session with the other counselor and in front of the couple. The counselor identified his concerns, and after careful review, decided that the issues might first need to be discussed in the Tandem Session before the individual session. While the counselors recovered from the procedural error, the need for consultation persisted. They eventually met with their supervisor and explored the fears that caused the un-expected response. They also developed a series of steps that they decided to use whenever one or the other member of the couple needed or asked for individual sessions. The steps included a clear way for all to communicate about the need for and the results of the individual meetings. This level of specificity helped not only the clients' re-lationship, but also the counselors'. High conflict couples can easily be triggered, so communication problems—especially sudden—are always disruptive, and therefore need to be avoided as much as possible.

A lack of congruence not only confuses clients, but also obstructs potential therapy gains. When two counselors have varying opinions about the clients' problems, diagnoses, strengths, and weaknesses, cli-ents can quickly sense and unwittingly use it against their own well-being. Because couples outwardly present in ways that can often mask their inner functioning—and the pathology—it can be very easy for one counselor to arrive at a vastly different diagnosis or level of concern from the other. The same is true for perceived strengths and weaknesses. One counselor may see one of the couple as more vulnerable than the other. These differences, if carefully managed, can be particularly useful during the therapy.

In this example one counselor considers the husband in a TCC couple to be very sturdy psychologically, and the other counselor sees him as quite frail. When discussing treatment alternatives, the counselors find themselves disagreeing about what to do next with the couple. One counselor feels the proposed intervention is warranted and necessary, while the other considers the intervention too risky and seriously be-yond the estimated ego strength of the husband. The counselors agree to remain open regarding the decision and spend a bit more time offering a basis for their opinions. The discussion leaves them wondering if they are talking about the same person since they have opposite outlooks. The counselors jointly decide to raise the difference of their opinions to the clients as a question for all of them to discuss. In session, they share that they have split views of the husband and cannot figure out why and ask the couple to make this a topic for them to discuss. The wife says, "I have been waiting to answer this question since we started dating almost 15 years ago!" The husband says, "I'm in because people always seem to see me as one way or the other, and I honestly do not know why." The counselors have now elevated a convergence problem into a valuable clinical exercise. In the end, the husband assertively says to his wife and his counselors, "I would like to be the one who decides whether I can and want to attempt something. All my life it has been others who choose for me as I either acted frailer than I really am or overly confident. It's time for me to honestly assess my strengths and weaknesses." Differences in opinion can be useful if they are openly discussed and allowed to evolve. On the other hand, when counselors react impulsively, the overall counseling effort is blunted—as with the case of countertransference.

Countertransference is a concept whose roots date back to psycho-analysis. The concept is a corollary to transference—redirecting feelings and reactions from an earlier relationship onto the therapist or counselor. In countertransference, the therapist redirects feelings and thoughts from a previous relationship onto a client. Despite the common perspective that countertransference is bad, "Countertransference is not, in and of itself, a problem, but how you react to these feelings can be" (Levitov & Fall, 2019, p. 72). TCC counseling sessions are susceptible to the same countertransference issues that are present in individual counseling as well as traditional couples counseling.

Our take on countertransference is both simple and unique; we believe that countertransference is an extremely useful force in counseling as long as it is "talked out" in the course of treatment rather than "acted out." The following individual counselor example may help to make the point clearer. Consider a client who exhibits a good deal of dependent behavior during his counseling sessions. His counselor is a woman who is the eldest of four siblings. During supervision, the counselor reveals that she had been asked to schedule a couple of extra sessions with her client because he was having difficulties at work and needed additional help. She also said that he had asked her to write a letter to his boss requesting that he get off work an hour earlier each day. She prepared the letter specifying that for health reasons, her client needed to end work at 4:00 PM instead of 5:00 PM but had not sent it. She said she felt a little funny about both requests but really wanted to help him as much as she could.

During supervision, the counselor was asked about the client's issues and the letter requesting an early leave time. The counselor surprised herself when she could not properly define a health problem she was aware of, which would justify the early leave time. She looked up quizzically and asked the supervisor, "Why did I do that?" Once a few more questions were answered the supervisor felt comfortable with the idea that a countertransference issue was lurking beneath the counselor's behavior. At this point, the supervisor empathically suggested that something other than the client's condition may be responsible for the counselor's choices and actions. Without so much as a moment's hesitation, the counselor said she had felt "funny" about the client from early in their clinical relationship. According to her, he reminded her of her youngest brother, the sibling that she had cared for when her mother became ill with a chronic health problem. The counselor realized that her reactions to her client were coming from a particularly important part of her own life and that she was not doing what she thought best for the client. The supervisor congratulated her on the insight and went about helping her with the issue she had correctly identified. The supervisor gently reminded her that acting on countertransference issues inhibits the counseling process while talking about these issues through improves the outcomes. The counselor shared how dependent her brother had become and how that dependence even felt good at times for her. She now had a firsthand understanding of the pattern of dependency that had been a part of her life and could now be easily observed in her clients. The supervisor then added, "You are in an enviable position to be helpful to your client because based upon your own life experiences, you understand the way dependency develops, how it actually works between two people, and the costs incurred." With one last question, the supervisor sought to help the counselor recover from the clinical concern: "What could you have done to talk out the reaction rather than act it out?" The counselor quickly answered, "I could have said to the client, 'I feel like you are asking me to do something for you, maybe you can try and do it for yourself. Can we talk about and explore your request, along with viable options?'" The following week during supervision, the counselor reported that the client had made such requests all of his life, and this was the first time he had a chance to consider the benefits and risks of living this way. He also asked, "What is it about me that encourages people to make decisions for me and take care of me?" She also knew exactly what to do with these two questions.

In TCC the countertransference issues surface from one or both counselors, and they can have the same negative effect on the therapy. Fortunately, in TCC there is always another professional in the rooms, so countertransference can be more easily identified with two sets of eyes studying each other's reactions. The resolution can also have a more profound effect because of TCC. When both counselors agree beforehand to address any countertransference concerns during in vivo consultations, the clients will have the benefit of observing how the issue is cooperatively identified and worked through by two professionals seeking to do the best for their clients. Since countertransference issues harken back to the counselor's family of origin and early life experiences, clients get to observe how those differences can be helpful when they are talked out rather than acted out.

In the previous TCC example, we discussed a lack of convergence among the counselors concerning the husband's psychological sturdiness. We can expand that same example as a useful description of counter- transference in a TCC setting. Let's modify the example to say that one counselor reacted very intensely during the counselors' outside meeting and became adamant about how frail he thought the husband actually was and decided that he would not participate in the foursome—where they would discuss the difference of opinion the counselors had come to. His reason: he believed that the client was indeed too frail to even have the question asked of him. The counselor then said that the Do No Harm clause in the Code of Ethics would prohibit questioning the husband at all. Surprised by the intensity of the co-therapist's remarks, the other counselor was left with more questions than answers. He decided that this level of intensity warranted the introduction of a third party, in this case, an experienced consultant. The other counselor agreed, and the duo scheduled the consult. During the consultation, it became obvious that there was more emotional intensity about the client's ego strength than seemed plausible. The consultant opened the possibility that the worried counselor was experiencing distress that was not justified within the setting. It did not take long for the distressed counselor to share some important elements about his father's psychological struggles and how his family had to be especially alert to make sure that his father did not become stressed. The counselor pursued some additional personal therapy to work through the attendant issues. He admitted that he deeply appreciated how gently his countertransference was handled by his clinical partner and their consultant. Countertransference issues are more easily detected and remedied in TCC; this counselor's personal issue could have been easily acted out with extremely negative consequences in another setting. Studying the effect countertransference has on the relationship between the counselors is always beneficial to the counselors and their clients. What might have been a serious dispute can become a source of deeper understanding and compassion for both the counselors and the couple.

Parallel Process is our way of thinking of a gold standard element for effective consultation and supervision. The underlying principle is both simple and powerful: whatever occurs in the context of the counseling relationship will replicate itself in the supervision or consultation interaction—this means patterns that occur when the counselor is working with their client will resurface in the supervision or consultation.

An example from a traditional, individual counseling session illustrates how a parallel process occurs and how valuable it is to training. Consider a counselor working with a client who has been struggling to make important life decisions. The counselor explains that it would be inappropriate for him to make decisions, but he is, nevertheless, committed to talking out options and possibilities. The client remains upset despite the explanation and then reacts bitterly towards the counselor by saying that he is very disappointed—that the therapy is doing nothing for him and, to make matters worse, it's costing a good deal of money. The counselor is uncertain what to do next and simply repeats the same points, making the client more frustrated and tells him it might be time to find a new counselor. Eventually, the counselor successfully encourages the client to schedule the meeting for next week and then tries to calm a bit, knowing he has a scheduled supervision meeting later that day.

During supervision, the counselor is obviously distressed. The counselor, almost immediately, confronts the supervisor with a host of complaints. He angrily tells the supervisor that supervision does not seem to be of much help. He complains that all they do is talk about "things" when what new counselors really need are extremely specific suggestions on what to say when various situations arise. He goes on to complain about the cost of supervision and the amount of time it takes to meet every week. Finally, the frustrated counselor asks, "Are there other supervisors out there who could better meet my professional needs?"

While you may think the example is overly fabricated, believe that such supervision sessions occur regularly, and they always resemble the counseling sessions the supervisee just completed. It is this amazing aspect of the parallel process that makes it so intensely useful to supervision and consultation. The rule: what happens between counselor and client will inevitably occur between counselor and supervisor-consultant. This process is often the lifeblood of supervision and consultation. Borders and Leddick captured the essence of the process in 1987 (p. 44) when they wrote, "Unable to verbally express all his/her perceptions of the client, the supervisee 'acts out' in an attempt to evoke in the supervisor the same feelings he/she experienced with the client (Hora, 1957)." After all these years, we both remain impressed by the frequency, intensity, and predictability of Parallel Process as well as intrigued by its usefulness. (For a more detailed description of Parallel Process please see Levitov and Fall [2019, pp. 60–72].)

In the noted example, the parallel process would be quickly addressed by any skilled supervisor or consultant. Once recognized (and appreciated) for what it is, the consultant or supervisor can easily label the activity, illustrate an empathic response to the counselor's frustration, appreciate the counselor's honest emotional reaction, and resolve the conflict. Fortunately, the resolution of the conflict also creates a clear and easy path for the counselor once he returns to the counseling session the following week—the counselor is now free to imagine what forces may have been at play to cause the client's reactions in the first place and develop better ways to manage them.

While parallel process is seen as productive to TCC, it is also complicated, and therefore easy to overlook if not focused on the relationship aspects of the work. Astute consultation or supervision is called for because the process can take on varied forms and more probable causes. Consider a couple in a TCC session struggling with parenting concerns. The husband always uses a more authoritarian stance with their children and urges his wife to do so as well; she disagrees and feels they need more support and understanding.

He claims that her position encourages the children to misbehave, but she feels his harshness makes the kids feel unloved and lonely. During the session, they pose the question of the best way to raise children to their TCC counselors. Uncertain about how to manage the emotional intensity surrounding the question, the counselors asked for an opportunity to complete an in vivo consultation about their next step—in no time, they also begin to argue about the best way to answer the couple's question. At this point, the wife interrupts and tells her husband that their couple's problem has now affected their counselors and confused them. Realizing the chaos that has ensued from the question and the counselors' awkward response, the counselors bring the process to a halt. One of the counselors admits that there really is not a conclusive answer to the question and creating more of a dispute is not helping. The session time runs out with all four participants confused and frustrated.

When TCC counselors gathered for their regular weekly supervision meeting, they immediately posed the parenting question to the supervisor. The supervisor correctly identified the feeling of being cornered and pressured to side with one of the counselors, and the inappropriate task of affirming that only one is correct. Having now experienced the projection emerging from the couple into the counselors and supervisor, they begin to understand what was happening. The supervisor responds empathically to the plight the counselors find themselves in and asks two questions: 1. "How did the clients' request affect your clinical/or professional relationship?" and 2. "How could your relationship respond more effectively to the client's conflict?" In the calm of the supervision setting, the counseling pair recognized that this was not an either-or but a both-and situation. The clients' children needed clear expectations for their behavior, appropriate consequences for misbehavior, as well as ample amounts of love and support from their parents. Eventually, both counselors admitted to the differences in the parenting styles each had experienced growing up and how unconsciously it found itself in the middle of their clinical work, judgment, and professional relationship.

What took more time to realize was the wife's uncanny insight into what was happening. One counselor mentioned just as they were preparing for the next meeting with the couple, "Did you catch that the wife actually identified the parallel process more accurately and more rapidly than we did?" The other's agreement spurred some further discussion. They eventually concluded that the wife had probably hoped for a more collaborative response, rather than the same ineffective pattern from which she and her husband suffered from, so she brought it to the counselors' attention. They agreed that they needed to make the client aware of what she had accomplished and thank her for her valuable insights. In the end, fears of being wrong, misunderstood, not taken seriously, and creating problems for their children all combined to saturate the counseling situation and overwhelm all participants. Contentedly, the analysis of the parallel process patterns restored stability and illuminated a proper path to resolution.

"Competent couples therapists evaluate not just the possibility but also the probability that interventions may inflict harm upon one or both members of the dyad" (Stratton & Smith, 2006, p. 342). In summary, reminding TCC counselors to be wary and vigilant about possible harm is critical. While there are many circumstances where such difficulties could emerge, we have discussed most of these areas in this section. By keeping all five in mind, and by the judicious use of supervisors and consultants, counselors can limit the risk of potential harm as they continuously improve their clinical relationship and expand their ability to help couples.

As we have stressed in TCC, the relationship between the therapists and the fruits of that relationship combine to heal the couple's relationship. We have illustrated what we think is added value resulting from two clinicians working together to help couples in distress. According to Breeskin, writing about group co-therapy (2013), "A single group therapist, no matter how skilled, cannot conceivably keep up with the richness of group experience. Important cues, particularly nonverbal ones, are in danger of being missed." The author also suggests that burnout becomes a very real possibility in groups where leadership is not shared. The author's conclusions are equally applicable to the couple's work. While seeing a couple is the smallest group setting possible, it remains, by definition, a form of group therapy. TCC, as a type of co-lead group therapy, offers many advantages. It is a protocol that can bind more anxiety, manage more chaos, resolve more conflict, and offer more support to clients than traditional approaches.

Under ideal conditions, TCC counselors should utilize co-therapy consultations on a regular basis and strive to seek outside supervision. We hope this section has prepared you for the process of consulting within the TCC framework. In the next section, we explore how to conduct the supervision of TCC in your training site or agency.

The Structure of Supervising TCC Counseling

The first part of the chapter was coming from the perspective of TCC practitioners and how they might utilize supervision in their work. This part of the chapter will focus on how to set up the supervision of TCC counselors and integrate the TCC approach into your training site. The information provided in the beginning will be helpful, but some additional elements might be useful in establishing a supervision component to your TCC journey.

It is assumed that the basics of supervision—supervisor training, ethical considerations, and other general matters—will already be integrated into your practice or training site. For an overview of the foundations of good supervision practice, we suggest Bernard and Goodyear (2018). More specifically, the following elements are considered critical when establishing a basis for effectively supervising TCC.

Assessing high conflict clientele: While TCC can be used with all relationship dyads, the genesis of the approach was to assist high conflict couples. Training centers, from a purely developmental perspective, might not be the best place to treat high conflict couples but TCC offers some inherent advantages to provide trainees, clients, and supervisors with added layers of support. Without TCC, training sites are left with two options—neither recommended. One is to refer clients under the concern that their dynamics and treatment needs exceed the level of expertise in the clinic. This decision can be disheartening for trainees and clients alike. Next, the site could assign the couple to more seasoned trainees and promise more intense supervision. However, due to the client's history and the intensity of the client interactions, it is probable that the trainees will be left overwhelmed—and the clients, dissatisfied. With TCC as an option, trainees are given a way to disperse the conflict across two counselors, process the patterns, and move toward relational growth while using the co-therapist and supervision relationship as a support structure. As mentioned in Chapter 2, having a way to assess high conflict is a necessary first step in considering the TCC option. Once the assessment model is in place, a pathway into TCC is established.

Developing a process for effective co-therapist pairing: The hallmark of the TCC approach is the use of the co-therapist relationship as an agent of change within the couple's work. Therefore, attention to appropriate co-therapist pairing is crucial. Many sources criticize the haphazard approach that many counselors use when forming co-therapy pairs, with the most common choice method being convenience (Berg, Landreth, & Fall, 2018; Roller & Nelson, 1991). We believe that the choice process must be deliberate and purposeful.

Training sites that are interested in employing the TCC approach should be mindful of these concerns and provide time and space for the exploration of possible co-therapy teams within their training groups. This can include the time when trainees spend time together in dyads or in a group, getting to know one another both professionally and personally. With co-therapy in mind, trainees can be encouraged to keep journals that remark their developing relationships with peers, noting the point of connection, and possible feelings of disconnect. As the relationships develop, supervisors create experiences where trainees can explore the areas of disconnect, noting how the trainees are managing the conflict. While this method does not have to be precisely followed, the point is that experiences need to be offered that allow both the supervisor and trainees the ability to focus and develop relationships with each other. These experiences will provide information into possible pairings that might effectively use the co-therapy relationship within TCC.

Establishing a consultation structure: The effort spent on quality assessment of high conflict couples and attention to developing healthy and productive co-therapy relationships will begin to show dividends within a consultation structure that encourages attention to both co-therapy and couple's dynamics. This is also the step where supervision begins to have a direct impact on the process, as supervision should be woven into the consultation process. In training agencies where trainees may be new to TCC, the structure will include both schedules for co-therapist consultation and supervision of the co-therapy team.

In the supervisory role, you should encourage the co-therapy team to meet at least weekly—before and after the session. A list of topics can be provided to help guide the discussion, keeping in mind that the purpose of the meetings is to improve the co-therapy relationship and focus on client conceptualization. A sample processing form is included in Table 7.1.

The team should also be meeting for weekly supervision. Much like traditional supervision, time can be allocated for feedback on counseling skills, the conceptualization of client issues, goal setting, and treatment planning. Unique to TCC will be the time that is focused on the quality of the co-therapy relationship. Supervisors must be skilled in illuminating the dynamics of the co-therapy relationship, providing insight into how the relationship could be used in the session, working through emerging obstacles in the co-therapy relationship, and paying attention to parallel process dynamics that occur during supervision. We realize that this is a lot to try to facilitate, but the process will be enhanced through quality supervision, and the stages of co-therapy relationship development outlined in Chapter 4 provide a good method to monitor progress.

Balancing client and co-therapist relationship conceptualization: We realize we covered the processing of both relationships—couple and co-therapist—in the last section, but the balance cannot be overstated. TCC requires the recognition and use of the co-therapy relationship in the change process of the couple. Monitoring the level of attention in these relationships can provide supervisors solid guidance regarding their state. For example, if the supervisor notices that the co-therapy team has neglected to meet with each other for a couple of weeks, it might be an indication that there is a disconnect in the relationship and would serve as a warning to bring this issue up in supervision. Good supervisors of TCC set up a structure for success that models the balance, but then must follow through on the actual practice of addressing all aspects of the relationships as the counseling progresses. A sample of supervision notes and a timeline is included in Table 7.2. We have found that this level of structure helps supervisors keep track of the various relational dynamics that are vital to the TCC process.

Using group supervision when possible: Group supervision is a required part of most mental health training programs and has been

Table 7.2 Sample Co-therapist Consultation Processing Form.

1 As I think about the consultation today, what am I feeling? How is this feeling
   reflected in my thoughts about the work of my client? About my co-therapist?
2 In thinking about my work with my client, what main patterns have emerged?
3 How internally focused is my client? How externally focused is my client?
4 As I think about the consultation today, what is one thing I want my co-therapist to
   know about my client? About me?
5 As I think about the consultation today, what is one thing that I want to learn about
   my client's partner? About my co-therapist?
6 How can I use the mindfulness elements of Investigation, Joy, Tranquility,
   Concentration, and Equanimity in the consultation today?

proven as an effective method of skill development and improvement
(Bostock, Patrizo, Godfrey, Munro, & Forrester, 2019; Kadushin &
Harkness, 2002; Munson, 2002). With group supervision so readily
available, supervisors must integrate this modality into their supervision
of TCC. Even if you only have a few trainees engaged in the TCC approach, the rest of the supervision group can learn the process indirectly
through the supervision process that occurs during the group.
Supervisors can also use the other trainees more actively by in-
corporating reflecting teams for the TCC teams, providing more feedback to the couple and trainees. For more on the use of reflecting teams,
consult Andersen (1991) or Reichelt and Skjerve (2013).

Modeling appropriate termination: Termination is important for
clients and therefore worth some attention in the co-therapy relationship. In fact, one of the advantages of the TCC approach is providing the
counselors with a termination processing venue of their own—namely
within the co-therapy relationship. While termination was discussed as
a stage of development in Chapter 4, supervision creates an ideal setting
to ensure the co-therapy team is processing termination within the
relationship and with the clients.

Supervisors should be aware of the following when processing termination within a TCC approach:

1   Each counselor's own pattern of saying good-bye in relationships;
2   Each client's patterns of saying good-bye in relationships; and

3   How the patterns noted above reflect other patterns in the work (both within the co-therapy and client relationships).

Having a sense of these allows the supervisor to illuminate the patterns and keep the counseling team aware while preparing for termination. This will ensure that the important dynamics are tended to and not avoided as the inherent anxiety associated with termination is experienced. It will also safeguard against the manifestation of dysfunctional responses to the anxiety, which could disrupt a safe and healthy termination. These problematic responses to termination—such as indifference, avoidance, anger, and helplessness—can often mirror client dynamics, so awareness and openness to parallel process elements can be helpful at this stage (Levitov & Fall, 2019). Where co-therapy teams are struggling with the process of termination, the termination of supervision can provide a useful model that can then be replicated with the co-therapy dyad. The following excerpt from a pre-termination meeting illustrates some of these dynamics and supervision can assist at the co-therapy and client levels.

Supervisor: Based on what you are telling me, it sounds like your clients are ready to complete their counseling.

Counselor 1:   I agree. I think they have done a wonderful job and have achieved what they came in to do.

Counselor 2:   We broached the subject last session, and they seemed a bit reluctant. Brooke got very anxious and said she was certain that they still had some things to work on. Dylan seemed a little miffed at that response but said he could see both sides of the issue.

Supervisor: How do those responses reflect their old patterns?

Counselor 2:   Good question. Brooke's tendency was to escalate conflict and worry that there was another problem around the corner: hypervigilance.

Counselor 1:   Yes, and Dylan typically responds by calling her crazy and acting like nothing was going on. At least some of the intense negativity was left out, but you can see the residual behaviors of that pattern.

Supervisor:	So, it might be helpful to point that out and refocus them on their new ways of handling that anxiety. Termination gives them one last opportunity to demonstrate their new skills! How are the two of you doing with the end of the co-therapy experience?
Counselor 1:	Oh, it's not the end. We will work together again, so there really isn't anything to discuss.
Counselor 2:	I am a little concerned that we haven't done enough for this couple. I mean, what if everything falls apart in the last session? Do we keep going?
Counselor 1:	Why would everything fall apart? They are doing great. I know we have a lot to learn, but we have time to do that with the next few cases we already have scheduled.
Supervisor:	I want us to take a moment here. Let's close our eyes and focus on the here and now, what's going on in the room, what is going on inside ourselves and between each other. Take a few deep breaths and open your eyes. What is in your immediate awareness of the moment?
Counselor 1:	As soon as I closed my eyes, I was first aware of my irritation with my co-therapist. I then focused on myself and realized that I was acting just like Dylan. I was responding to her anxiety by trying to whisk it away.
Counselor 2:	That's so cool. I was aware of my irritation with you for glossing over the termination. I thought, "That's just like him to ignore the importance of what we are talking about," but then I realized I didn't really feel that way about you. It was Brooke talking to Dylan. I didn't feel like you were taking me seriously and that is the root of disrespect in their relationship.
Supervisor:	Well done. You have identified some powerful patterns. How do you want to handle them, both for your relationship and the clients?
Counselor 2:	I think this will help us be prepared for how they might respond to the termination; we got a glimpse of that

last session. I'm a little worried that Brooke might feel abandoned and if Dylan suggests not showing up, that they might not show for the last session.

Counselor 1:   We should call our respective clients, foreshadow this possibility, and reinforce the importance of the last session. What about our relationship?

Counselor 2:   Well, as I said, it's weird because we will be working on other cases.

Supervisor: But this is the end of this part of the relationship. Think of your time together as a book and this is the end of the chapter. How do you want to honor the end of this part and the work you have done?

Counselor 2:   I see what you mean. I hadn't thought of it like that. I think it would be nice to meet after the session and process the work. Talk about what we learned about ourselves, each other, the workings of TCC.

Counselor 1:   I like that idea. We can highlight the things we thought worked and things we want to do differently moving forward.

This dialogue illustrates how supervision can be utilized to identify helpful patterns within the co-therapy relationship and assist the co-therapists in the application of those patterns into their work with clients. In this example, termination issues were explored, both in terms of client development and its impact on the co-therapy team. The awareness of and attention to these interwoven dynamics is the essence of good supervision and the hallmark of what is needed to make the most of the TCC approach.

Summary

We both share great enthusiasm and respect for the processes of supervision and consultation. As students, we honestly looked forward to obtaining as much supervision from many different supervisors possible; as teachers, we always look forward to working with supervisees and consultees; and as practicing clinicians, we remain actively involved in both peer and individual consultation. Ironically, students regularly assumed that we knew "enough," so they were always surprised when they find out that we had never worked without consultation—and we never would no matter how long we practiced. We realized, early in our training that there is always something new to learn, and a chance we might miss something important that only a third party could help find. TCC supervision for us is another exciting journey, one filled with interesting possibilities and unique opportunities. We hope that you will obtain skilled TCC supervision-consultation as you explore the principles and methods shared in this text. We also hope that you will consider exploring ways you can contribute by supervising or consulting with others as they apply TCC. Such efforts to help couples find intimacy, peace, and happiness in their relationships—as well as the relationships around them—are worthwhile and critically important.

References

Andersen, T. (1991). *The reflecting team: Dialogues and dialogues about the dialogues.* Boston: Norton.

Berg, R. C., Landreth, G. L., & Fall, K. A. (2018). *Group counseling: Concepts and procedures* (6th ed.). New York: Routledge.

Bernard, J. M., & Goodyear, R. (2018). *Fundamentals of clinical supervision* (6th ed.). New York: Pearson.

Borders, L. D., & Leddick, G. R. (1987). *Handbook of counseling supervision.* Alexandria, VA: Association for Counselor Education and Supervision.

Bostock, L., Patrizo, L., Godfrey, T. T. G., Munro, E. E., & Forrester, D. F. (2019) How do we assess the quality of group supervision? Developing a coding framework. *Children & Youth Services Review, 100*, 515–524.

Bradley, L. J., Ladany, N., Hendricks, B., Whiting, P. P., & Rhode, K. (2010). Overview of counseling supervision. In N. Landry & L. J. Bradley (Eds.), *Counselor Supervision* (4th ed., pp. 3–13). New York: Routledge.

Breeskin, J. (2013). The co-therapist model in groups: Four reasons why group therapists should not administrate group sessions independently. *Adult Development and Aging News 23*(1), 7–8.

Kadushin, A., & Harkness, D. (2002). *Supervision in social work* (4th ed.). New York: Columbia University Press.

Levitov, J. E., & Fall, K. A. (2019). *Becoming an effective counselor: A guide for advanced clinical courses.* New York: Routledge.

Munson, C. E. (2002). *Handbook of clinical social work supervision* (3rd ed.). New York: Haworth Social Work Practice Press.

Reichelt, S., & Skjerve, J. (2013). The reflecting team model used for clinical group supervision without clients present. *Journal of Marital & Family Therapy, 39*(2), 244–255.

Roller, B., & Nelson, V. (1991). *The art of co-therapy: How therapists work together.* New York: Guilford Press.

Stratton, J. S., & Smith, R. D. (2006). Supervision of couples cases. *Psychotherapy, Research, Practice, Training, 43*(3), 337–348.

INDEX

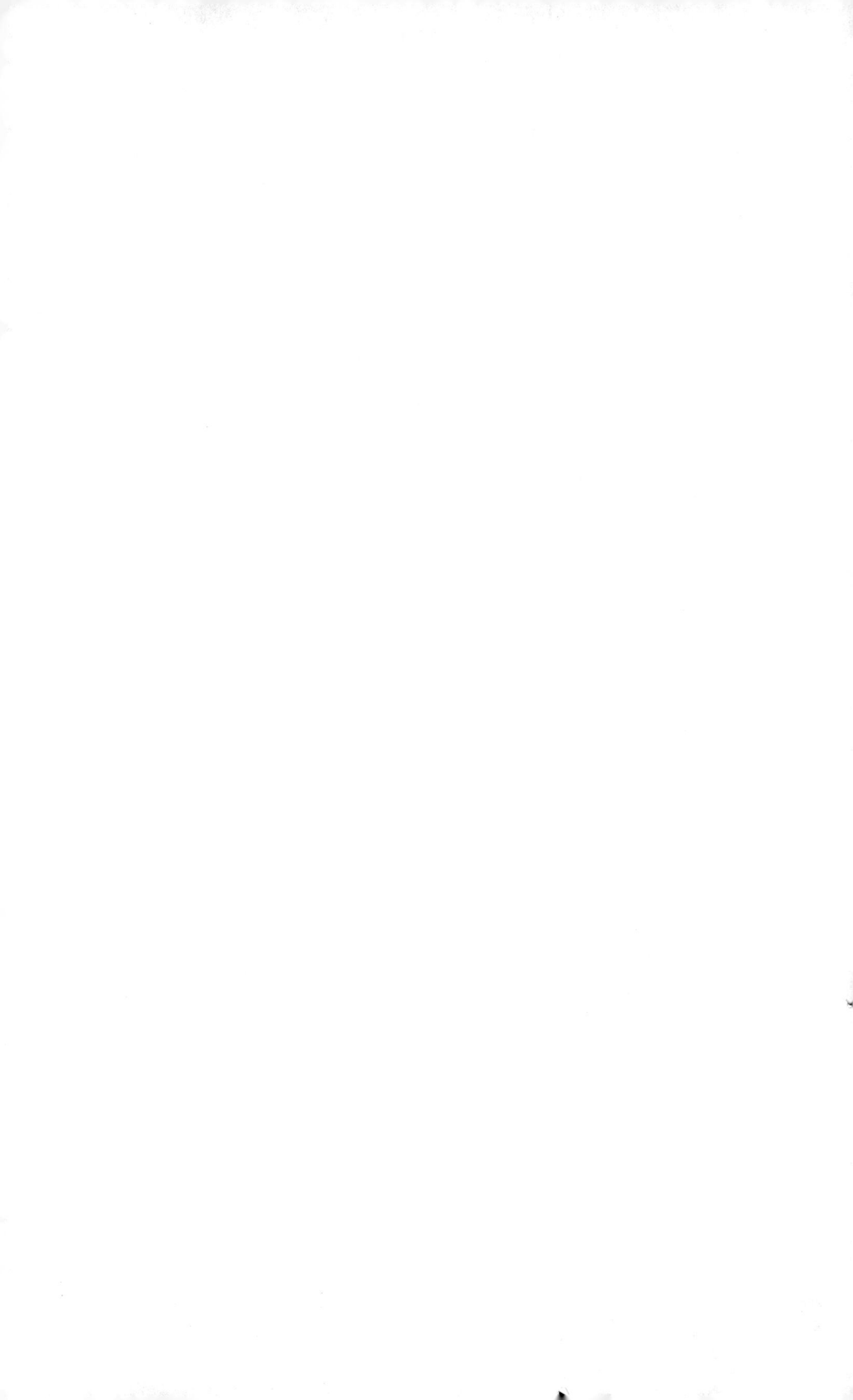

For Product Safety Concerns and Information please contact our EU
representative GPSR@taylorandfrancis.com
Taylor & Francis Verlag GmbH, Kaufingerstraße 24, 80331 München, Germany